IN

We dedicate this book to special family members who have seen us through life changes: Lyn to her mother and father; Carmel to her mother; Nicki to her brother, Craig.

INTERMISSION
WOMEN, MENOPAUSE AND MIDLIFE

LYN RICHARDS

CARMEL SEIBOLD

NICOLE DAVIS

Melbourne
OXFORD UNIVERSITY PRESS
Oxford Auckland New York

OXFORD UNIVERSITY PRESS AUSTRALIA
Oxford   New York
Athens   Auckland   Bangkok   Bombay
Calcutta   Cape Town   Dar es Salaam   Delhi
Florence   Hong Kong   Istanbul   Karachi
Kuala Lumpur   Madras   Madrid   Melbourne
Mexico City   Nairobi   Paris   Port Moresby
Singapore   Taipei   Tokyo   Toronto
and associated companies in
Berlin   Ibadan

OXFORD is a trade mark of Oxford University Press

© Lyn Richards, Carmel Seibold, Nicole Davis 1997
First published 1997

This book is copyright. Apart from any fair dealing for the purposes of private study, research, criticism or review as permitted under the Copyright Act, no part may be reproduced, stored in a retrieval system, or transmitted, in any form or by any means, electronic, mechanical, photocopying, recording or otherwise without prior written permission. Enquiries to be made to Oxford University Press.

Copying for educational purposes
Where copies of part or the whole of the book are made under Part VB of the Copyright Act, the law requires that prescribed procedures be followed. For information, contact the Copyright Agency Limited.

National Library of Australia
Cataloguing-in-Publication data:

Richards, Lyn 1944-.
  Intermission: women's experiences of menopause and mid-life.
  Includes index.
  ISBN 0 19 553947 8.
  1. Menopause - Popular works. 2. Middle aged women - Health and hygiene. I. Seibold, Carmel.
  II. Davis, Nicole. III. Title.
612.665

Edited by Katherine Steward
Cover design by Steve Randles
Typeset by Derrick I Stone Design
Printed by Kin Keong, Singapore
Published by Oxford University Press,
253 Normanby Road, South Melbourne, Australia

Contents

1	Introduction *Lyn Richards*	1
2	Women's images of menopause *Nicole Davis*	13
3	Mirrors of menopause — the popular literature *Carmel Seibold and Nicole Davis*	32
4	The body in midlife *Carmel Seibold*	48
5	Making the Change *Lyn Richards*	77
6	One woman's story *Mary Fisher*	105
7	Private parts in public places *Nicole Davis, Carmel Seibold and Lyn Richards*	126
8	Natural and unnatural risk — midlife and women's health *Claire Parsons and Val Seeger*	149
9	What *did* the doctor say? *Lyn Richards*	171
10	Another sort of care? Community level advice *Lyn Richards*	199
	Postscript	226
	List of information and support services	229
	Notes	230
	References	233
	Index	240

1
INTRODUCTION

Lyn Richards

This is a book about women's midlives. It began as a research project to study menopause as a socially constructed experience. It became a study of midlife because women made it so; when we asked about menopause, they talked about all the processes of life changes in the middle years. It then became a study of the multiplicity of midlives, as the variety of women's experiences became evident. It started, directed by the literature, as a study of transition: the ways in which women's lives are irrevocably altered by 'the Change' of menopause and the other changes of midlife. Women's accounts forced us to rethink the assumptions we had brought from our reading, our personal backgrounds and our societal stereotypes, to see midlife and menopause not as transition (becoming something different, and less desirable) but as an interval, a time when women, in many different ways, take or are overtaken by a break in the performance of their lives. Late in the process of analysis we decided to rename this book. Menopause, we concluded, was not the drama but the *intermission*, the pause in a continuing performance.

MAKING DATA

This book is also the outcome of an adventure in teamwork and marathon data analysis. The project, which had been funded for three years from 1991 to 1993,[1] was designed to create unique data, and it did. Lots of unique data! The proposal was to develop an interpretative framework for understanding the range of women's perceptions and experiences of menopause as a complex interaction between social and cultural phenomena, and their physiological base. 'Qualitative' data, made by recording women's own words and our observations, was to be studied in detail. 'Quantitative' data from a survey was to be statistically analysed. The two sorts of data were to be combined, linked by the use of qualitative computing (Richards & Richards 1995).

Few projects, and particularly few qualitative projects, go according to plan, and researchers are often constrained from admitting the difficulties encountered. In this project, the original design proved highly problematic. Consistent with tenets of qualitative method, techniques of data collection and analysis were data-driven and responded to early research stages.

Group interviews

In the first year, 1991, nine group interviews (including a total of about 100 women) highlighted a set of issues to be pursued, but also a set of problems with the method. Volunteer samples showed a bias towards middle-class experience and, worse, the groups reflected the bias of researchers. Individual speakers were hard to identify in transcripts, which gave little sense of the context of a woman's experience. Group interviewing also raised serious ethical issues: an intrusive and sometimes manipulative method, it benefited articulate women. Some participants later reported they had felt uncomfortable and were unable to speak easily of their experience or had felt 'bullied' by the group (especially into taking a critical stance against the 'biomedical perspective' on the issue of hormone replacement therapy or HRT). Qualitative data from individual interviews, by contrast, indicated women's experiences should be studied as contextualised processes, of body and identity changes and what we later termed 'transition work' (see chapter 5). Group interviews were discontinued in this project sector, and sampling and interviewing methods were varied to ensure a spread of socio-economic status and geographical location and to seek fuller accounts from a wider range of women in more varied settings by more varied methods.

STUDY OF SINGLE WOMEN

Meanwhile, Carmel Seibold had commenced her study of twenty single women's experiences of midlife and menopause. Her very detailed private interviews were gathering a quite different picture of the complexity and nuances of women's experiences, and the diaries kept by these women showed the intensity of experience and rapidity of change. Understanding of the process was to be enhanced by a second interview a year later.

PHONE INTERVIEWS WITH HEALTH PROVIDERS

As issues of trust and authority of medical knowledge emerged as significant themes in women's accounts, it became evident that we needed to find out more about the health advice being offered. We started with health providers at community level, since the messages from that level were about 'holistic' care and oppositon to the 'narrow' biomedical approach. We phoned each community health centre or citizen's advice bureau in Melbourne, and talked to someone in each place (eighty-five in total) where we were told advice was given on menopause. The telephone interviews were brief but provided insight into the assumptions and responses of people who act as information gatekeepers for women. The data firmly rebutted arguments in the literature that all nurses have a single perspective on this issue, and gave us a vivid picture of the community level of care, and the messages women hear there.

POPULAR LITERATURE AND MAGAZINE REVIEWS

We reviewed the discussion of menopause in popular books and magazines around the period of our study, from 1986 to 1992.

We found a most unexpected variety of images and advice concerning medical approaches.

REACHING OUT — THE AREA STUDIES

In the second year, the present team discarded the group-interview format, and set out to locate a wider range of experiences, to provide more private settings for women to talk, and to identify what women did hear from medical authorities and what doctors and other health providers were trying to say. Contrasting area studies were designed to offer a range of settings and experiences. On the basis of census maps, we selected five local government areas of Melbourne and its rural environs that would offer contrasts on demographic profile, indicators of socio-economic status, women's education and ethnic diversity.

Studies of these local areas combined background research, field research and interview data to enable us to place women's accounts within a detailed picture of the demographic and social setting, and to establish the medical, alternative medical and paraprofessional resources available in an area, and the social networks, opportunities and resources for sharing experience and information. The range of women's situations and experiences across the areas proved very considerable, offering rich and detailed data on the pathways of women into different responses and experiences, and the approaches to community-level information taken in different areas. We used a range of methods for finding and listening to women, including participant observation at groups and community houses, contacts with general practitioners, alternative health professionals and counsellors, local publicity for the project and publicising requests for women to contact us. By these methods we built up large bodies of data in field notes and taped individual interviews. To some extent this rectified the middle-class bias of volunteer samples, but both the survey and the qualitative data overrepresent middle-class women. Given no funding for translators, we made no attempt to represent non-English-speaking women.

In each area, first contacts were made by phone and in person with community groups and health providers, snowball contacts were followed to interview those involved in organising or participating in groups for midlife women. Women were sought through information sheets given out by health providers and placed in libraries, waiting rooms, and other places where they may have been seen (coffee lounges, chemists etc.). We offered women four ways of contributing to the project: talking on the phone, writing to us, answering a questionnaire, or doing a face-to-face interview. Many women spoke eagerly and with interest about midlife and menopause, most women interviewed had shared their experiences with others, albeit often with embarrassment. Most women knew the subject was widely aired in the media. Eighty face-to-face interviews were conducted with women contacted by these means. We were, however, also keen to reach women who did not meet in groups or discuss issues of menopause in public. 'Written interview' questionnaires were designed, with informal formatting and presentation, and sent to women who wished to contribute but were unhappy about personal interviews or discussions (seventy were returned). These questionnaires piloted the survey questionnaire that was developed later. Twenty face-to-face interviews and ten questionnaire interviews were conducted with general practitioners and alternative health providers in the five areas.

A WIDER PICTURE — THE LARGE-SCALE SURVEY

To these pictures of individual women's experiences, we provided a backdrop sketch of wider societal attitudes. A random sample was drawn of all adult women in the five areas, linking the survey methodologically and in background to the previous area studies. Questionnaires were sent to 3000 women. Given the highly sensitive subject matter, the likely irrelevance of midlife issues to a large proportion of the target population, and the high address-unknown return rate in the semi-rural areas, a low response rate was expected. The initial response rate of nearly one third was encouraging, and the returns showed a large proportion of open-ended responses. Follow-up telephoning of a random selection of the total sample resulted in a final return of 1069 questionnaires, well spread across age groups and areas.

SURVEYING ON A SENSITIVE ISSUE

There is a substantial groundswell of social sciences opinion opposing survey research on sensitive issues, health issues and women's issues. This literature was considered very seriously in the design and conduct of the survey. Substantial attention was given to the design of the 'written interview' style questionnaire, to encourage open-ended responses. The ethical challenges of surveying were seriously addressed: a 'hotline' phone was staffed for two weeks during the survey, and telephone follow-ups were done by women. Recipients of the questionnaire and of later follow-up calls were assured that the survey was anonymous. To validate this assurance, the normal practice of marking and recording returns to a survey was not followed. It is worth noting that several women told us they were impressed by this, justifying the extra expense of being unable to target follow-up calls to those who had not responded. Women we phoned who had already responded were uniformly positive about the experience, and impressed and reassured by the evidence that we had not identified their forms. Experience with this survey suggests that the critical attack on surveying should be directed towards insensitive survey approaches, rather than blanket dismissal of quantitative research methodology.

The data are of course limited by the brevity of the questionnaire. Nevertheless the questionnaires offered a different, totally anonymous and safe way in which women could contribute. They may misrepresent women's responses less seriously than the often threatening context of an intimate group discussion or in-depth interview. This is not to argue that concerns about superficial or offensive impersonal research methods should be dismissed, or to discount the methodological imperative behind high-quality qualitative research, of understanding the complexity and context of experience. Rather, the experience of this project suggests that a combination of approaches, if the data can be rigorously combined, may best address the complexity of a subject and the ethical considerations of respondents' needs.

ASKING NEW QUESTIONS — THE RISK PERCEPTION PROJECT

As our understanding of the data developed, so too did our awareness of questions our data could not answer. Central was the emerging theme of risk. How and when was midlife and menopause equated with risk? It seemed that women were having midlife and menopause defined for them as risky, by an odd collaboration of medical and feminist discourses, where hitherto it had been a natural stage of life. HRT had become the issue for many women we interviewed, and their discussions of it were dominated by concern that they were at risk whether or not they took it. Discussions with Claire Parsons, who had worked on risk in medical contexts, led to a piggy-back project funded in 1994–95. This time our approach was more structured, as we knew the questions we wanted to ask. Val Seeger asked them of 167 women, 35 to 60 years of age, who were selected by random sampling in the same five areas as the main project. The women's answers were recorded on tape.

HANDLING THE DATA

The goals were to provide rigorous qualitative analysis, and to combine qualitative and quantitative data. All qualitative data records were coded using qualitative software I co-designed (the QSR NUD•IST software for Non-numerical Unstructured Data Indexing, Searching and Theorising). The survey data were handled in SPSS and integrated with qualitative analysis in QSR NUD•IST by use of command files to input data from one data preparation process into both packages (Richards 1996).

The QSR NUD•IST program permitted rigorous processing of the unusually large amount of qualitative data required by the research design. The software allowed linking of the varied types and sources of qualitative data for comparison and synthesis. It had huge implications for team research, allowing communication between members and collaboration on development of ideas, but also threatened the team by highlighting differences in computer competence and fear of computers. We've written about these problems elsewhere (Richards 1995) and urge other teams to talk honestly about the challenges faced when moving into the new technologies now supporting qualitative research.

Our managing to report on large-scale qualitative data should not be taken as an argument for large-scale projects unless the topic requires them. The volume of our data proved formidable, and the need to balance organisation and creativity was a major challenge. Routinisation of analytical tasks always threatened as data built up faster than it could be analysed.

WHAT DID WE FIND?

Our data challenged simple assumptions about midlife and menopause in every way. In particular it rebuked three of the most widely accepted assertions about menopause: that menopause is taboo, experienced in secret; that women experience menopause as a dreaded transition, from desired femininity and youth to despised old age; and that medical advice is constrained to a narrow, scientific 'biomedical' perspective.

We found that women's experiences of midlife were strongly set in social images of ageing and femininity. However the data provided no simple picture of women's experience dictated by these social images. Chapter 2 shows there is no fixed, dominant image, rather that images are constructed in the interplay between social context and experience. Images are patterned by age group, appearing and fading in different age groups. There was no evidence for the usual stereotypes of menopause: taboo, sick, ill, curable. The rest of this book is about the ways women actively construct their understandings. While images of menopause were overwhelmingly negative, the subject is certainly not now taboo.

When we reviewed the popular sources of information, books and magazines (see chapter 3) we found that the HRT story dominated in the early 1990s, but that interest appeared to decrease later. We found little evidence of two competing models, biomedical and holistic, rather that the literature contained many models, and none unchanging.

We learnt from women's accounts about their relationships with their changing bodies. Chapter 4 draws on the single-women study, which showed women working the body, in the public context of work and the private context of role and obligations; controlling the body by control of fertility (and by implication sexuality) and by controlling menopause with HRT; listening to the body, developing 'in tune' relationships with the changing body; and viewing the body.

We learnt that our assumption that we were studying a transition, 'the Change' of a woman from one state to another, was almost always unfounded. As chapter 5 explains, it took us a long time to realise how unsatisfactory the metaphor of transition is for the experience of most midlife women. We brought from popular literature and feminist debates the expectation that in our data menopause and midlife would be transition. We found transitions, and learnt about transition work — the ways some women make and manage change at midlife. However, we slowly came to the conclusion that menopause is a clear transition for very few women, and they are generally the ones who choose to make it so. All women experienced some sense of change, temporary or permanent. But their experiences varied enormously, and very few were of transition. Rather, what women seemed to experience in common was an intermission, interruption, sometimes minimal, sometimes critically serious, in their lives.

We learnt from the women's detailed accounts of how agonising and enthralling the experience can be, how 'time out' from routine existence can make the intermission one of reflection and revival, and how active some women can be in constructing and directing the next act of the drama. Chapter 6 offers the story of one woman's experience, told through her diary entries over one year.

We learnt a lot about contexts: women's experiences could be understood only when they were seen as happening somewhere. Work — paid work — was shown as central. We found that for many in this generation of women, paid work is the crucial setting for experience of midlife. People in the survey had strong views about the effect of paid work on menopause and midlife. Women's stories in each chapter tell of the range of experiences for which work was the setting: excruciatingly embarrassing, highly positive, exhausting, confirming. We learnt about wider contexts, and particularly the social and geographical location of women's experiences and the relevance of distance, social and physical. Chapter 7 explores these contexts through the stories of five women in very different situations, concluding that the ways women experience change, vulnerability and support, ignorance and advice, fear and confidence, were not determined, but mediated by these contexts.

We learnt of the sense of danger and risk that women felt, often with distress, concerning menopause. This issue is explored in chapter 8. Menopause was seen as offering an unnatural risk as opposed to 'natural' disease. Anxiety about the decision whether or not to accept hormone treatment was high, and women often expressed relief if this decision was taken away from them by authoritative medical instruction. Concern about risk seemed to have little relationship to preventative or screening behaviour and interpretations of screening gave grounds for concern. The messages received from health promotion campaigns, that women are responsible for their health, proved to be a heavy burden.

How do health providers contribute to these constructions? The project had been proposed in the context of critical dogma about the 'biomedical perspective', its hostility to women and its uniformly medical interpretations of their experience. Much of our data challenged these assumptions. As chapter 9 shows, health providers' perceptions and interpretations were shown to be complex social constructions. While this data justifies concern about the ways in which women are advised and the sources of medical knowledge, there was little evidence that medical advice was dictated by 'positivist' textbook knowledge. Women's stories challenged simple assumptions that doctors uniformly apply a narrow biomedical perspective to issues of women's health. While an ideal type of biomedical interpretation of menopause was identified, few accounts from women or professionals fitted this type. Professionals' responses ranged from unquestioned recommendation of hormone treatment, through more varied or 'holistic' care, to anxiety and uncertainty about appropriate responses.

We were thus led to explore other sources of medical knowledge, and to discuss critically the myths and unintended results of the commitment at community level to health advice for women. Chapter 10 reports on this other sort of care, and finds it different, but not in the ways represented in the community health literature. Menopause is portrayed as an issue of public health, women are told to be responsible for their health and are prepared by instruction on a wide range of debilitating possible conditions — the messages at the local level were sometimes depressing and worrying.

WHERE DID WE COME FROM — AND GET TO?

This book is the construction of many women, not just the authors. Most obviously, our understanding is based on the stories told to us by around 2000 women who participated in different parts of the project. While no real names have been used, the book is made up of their voices. We thank them all, and hope that some of them see this book and many hear about it, and that those who do will tell us what they think of it and continue the discussions we started with them. We learned from them, laughed with them, sympathised with them and admired them, were angered, depressed, elated, excited, awed and inspired by their stories. The data constantly overwhelmed us and still does.

The data making and handling involved many other women

who do not appear as authors, and who of course are not responsible for what we have written. Cathi Lewis worked on the Mornington Peninsula study throughout the project. Others were part of it for a shorter time. In the first year, Jeanne Daly was a co-principal researcher and Freya Headlam conducted a literature review. For two years, Dawn Simon was senior research assistant; she also conducted some interviews with health providers, as did Heather Jarman. Amanda Jenkins reviewed magazines and attended groups. Cathy Maisano coded qualitative and survey data. Linda Salomons was a visiting associate, interviewing women and doctors. Maureen Greed and Irene Am interviewed women in distant areas, and Maureen attended a series of group information sessions. Lynne Ruggiero and Shelley Gooch typed interview transcripts. Peter Davidson, our token male, joined the team to assist with the survey.

The authors were also actors in the construction of the data. We introduce ourselves in the chapters to come as we write of the data we helped construct, which affected our own understanding of our lives. All of us found it changed our ideas on ideological portrayals of women and their treatment by health providers. As feminists we rethought the accepted critical stance as we recognised women's agency and the complexity of their experiences. So you will find no simple party line in this book. If we share a position now, it is that women are neither the mindless puppets of societal images, nor victims of a male biomedical conspiracy, but that critical awareness of their material and ideological context is essential to understanding what they themselves make of their lives during midlife.

2
WOMEN'S IMAGES OF MENOPAUSE

Nicole Davis

Women's experiences of family and health at midlife are influenced by social images of ageing and femininity. But how set are these images? Do women of all age groups have similar perceptions of midlife? How has each generation interpreted society's presentation of midlife? For a broader picture of Australian women's images of midlife, women aged 18 and above were surveyed. The survey was to provide a backdrop, a wider picture of societal attitudes, to the more detailed accounts of women's experiences that had been gathered during our two years of interviewing a range of women. The survey drew on these accounts, allowing us to explore how general the images and concerns we had heard from particular women were.

For me all of what women said about midlife and menopause was new. I was in my early twenties and had not even thought about having children let alone any life stage which followed. I shared the experience of discovering what midlife and menopause meant to many Australian women with my fellow researcher, Cathy Maisano. We worked together to send out and then organise the numerous survey responses. We joked that all our knowledge about menopause and midlife would make us very paranoid 40-year-olds.

The research team approached the survey with concern. We wanted to ask women about experiences, expectations and images of midlife and menopause, their sources of information and health care, and whether they thought society's attitudes were changing. We didn't know what to expect. The topic was potentially embarrassing and personal, and probably of little interest to younger women and older women. Would anyone respond to an impersonal questionnaire on such a subject? If they did respond, would they tell us anything we did not already know from our long, detailed interviews with other women?

They did respond and they told us a lot. The survey showed midlife and menopause located in a range of complex images — it gave us a chance to view patterns of change across age groups and provided us with a sense of how images are mediated by experience and knowledge.

This chapter begins by reporting on how the data were collected and analysed. A picture of the women who responded to the survey is included, and their images of midlife and perceptions of society's attitudes to midlife are also explored.

Designing the survey

The data were drawn from a random sample of adult women in five very different local government areas (Kew, Preston, Werribee, Frankston and Mornington) in Melbourne, between December 1992 and February 1993. Three thousand surveys were mailed out. Considering the delicate topic, we were delighted that 1069 were finally returned. To improve the response rate we had telephoned a random sample of the women three weeks after the mailing to encourage them to complete the survey. As the follow-up telephone calls were based on a random sample, some of those telephoned had already completed the questionnaire. This reassured the women who had returned their survey that their responses were truly confidential and that we did not hold any information which could identify them. Anonymity was promised and we guaranteed that promise by having no identification on the surveys we sent out.

During the weeks of the survey we staffed a 'hotline' phone number to discuss and explain our project. Only four calls were negative, two were from husbands expressing their concern that their partners were contributing personal information. We explained to them that all responses were anonymous.

The questionnaire was developed in several stages. An earlier version was sent to women who did not wish to be interviewed as part of the area study. We experimented with ways of presenting questions as a 'written interview'. Questionnaires were set out in an open format with generous amounts of space to invite women to comment, not just circle responses. The final questionnaire had an open format and was almost too successful. Women wrote extensively and provided us with long, open-ended comments. Often they attached pages to the end of the survey. To our alarm we realised that our survey had created qualitative data, in considerable bulk. This sort of data, over a thousand questionnaires all containing qualitative and quantitative responses, could not possibly be analysed without specialist computer programs. The quantitative data was analysed using SPSS while the qualitative data was analysed using NUD•IST, linked to SPSS via NUD•IST command files (for a full discussion see Richards 1995).

The women who returned the surveys were from a wide range of backgrounds and age groups. We set out to develop a picture of all women's images of midlife and how these images are changing. The data defied simple interpretation. It taught us to question many of the stereotypes in the literature, and to reconsider what the women had told us in their interviews.

Respondents' family, cultural and economic context

We expected Australian-born women to be overrepresented in our sample as the questionnaire was in English, which would impede responses from some overseas-born women. Even though the majority of women were born in Australia, thirty-eight other countries of birth were also nominated.

All of us anticipated a low response rate among younger women, assuming that they would have a lack of interest in the topic. But our age distribution was skewed towards younger and older women. The distribution of age groups seemed an indicator of our success at developing a survey to which all women would feel their responses were relevant. A review of all five-year age-group breaks indicated that slightly more women aged under 30 (15%) returned the survey. Women aged over 70 comprised the second highest response group (14%).

Of the women surveyed, 24% were aged between 31 and 40 and 17% were aged between 41 and 50. The number of women aged between 51 and 60 was 13%, and between 61 and 70, 17%.

Like the population of Australian women, our sample consisted largely of women who were married or cohabiting adults (65%). Similar to the Australian statistics for women living alone at this time (20%), 18% of the women in our sample lived by themselves.[1] Forty-five per cent had children living at home, with the majority (32%) having two children. Most of the women lived in households where the average yearly income was under $50 000: for 39% it was under $25 000 a year and for 35% it was under $50 000.

Just under half of all the women surveyed were in paid work. Twenty-five per cent were in part-time work, while 23% were in full-time employment. Of the women surveyed 38% were not employed and not wanting to be. Eleven per cent of women surveyed were seeking some form of paid employment.

A slight majority of employed women worked in the clerical area (12%), while 10% of women surveyed were either professionals or worked in the sales and service industries. Para-professional employment accounted for 6% surveyed.

Respondents' health and health care

We had expected our research topic to be of more interest to those women whose health was a concern to them. However, as the following information indicates, the health status of women who responded covered a wide range.

HEALTH AND FITNESS

Women overwhelmingly described their current health as good (49%) or very good (30%). Only three women described their present health as very poor. Nearly all of the women surveyed said being fit was important to them (important 47%, very important 39%). The majority exercised regularly, either weekly (22%) or more often than weekly (36%). Seven per cent of women never exercised and 34% exercised only occasionally. Given the high number of older women who responded, these figures differ strikingly from the Australian Bureau of Statistics (1993) report that 16.7% of Australian women exercised at a medium rate, while only 11.8% were high exercisers. The question is, of course, one that people like to respond to favourably.

GYNAECOLOGICAL HISTORY

Of the 1069 women surveyed 162 had had a hysterectomy. Six others were uncertain whether they had had a hysterectomy, an alarming indication of poor communication between them and their doctors. Seventy-four of these women had had their ovaries removed (13 were uncertain). Women who had had a hysterectomy were asked how it affected their health: 108 felt it had improved their health, 31 felt it had no effect, 11 perceived it had worsened their health, and 23 had mixed feelings. (A minority of the women circled two of these responses, hence they add up to more than 162.)

SCREENING

A high proportion of women reported that they actively participated in health prevention through screening. The tests women reported having in the past five years for health screening are illustrated in Table 2.1. We do not know which tests were self initiated and which were done at the request of doctors. The figures also indicate that 26% of the women said that they should have had a health-screening test but had not, of these 23% cited a pap smear and 37% a mammogram.

Table 2.1 Health-screening

Health-screening test	Tests taken % of women surveyed	Test not taken but should be % of those who said they not taken tests they should take
Mammogram	22	37
Pap smear	64	23
Cholesterol	32	14
Bone-density scan	5	9
X-ray	5	—
Colonoscopy	9	—
Ultrasound	19	—
Blood tests	33	6
Cat scan	7	—
All others	36	11

Note: Some women circled more than one test.

USE OF PROFESSIONALS

Women were asked who they sought health advice from. Not surprisingly the majority of the sample went to a doctor (92%). To investigate the prevalence of women shopping around for health advice we asked them if they went to the same health professional for all their consultations: 61% did and 39% attended a range of health professionals. Even though women nominated doctors as someone they seek health advice from, many also reported seeking advice from a range of other practitioners, including physiotherapists (25%), masseurs (7%), cardiologists (6%), dentists, Chinese medicine specialists and kinesiologists (these answers nominated thirty-two different types of practitioners).

MENOPAUSAL STATUS OF RESPONDENTS

The majority of the sample (46%) reported that they were before menopause while 35% had finished menopause. Four per cent of the women were starting menopause, 8% were in menopause, and 6% were uncertain of their status. We also asked women how sure they were of the stage they were in: 6% were unsure, 29% were fairly sure and the majority of women (67%) were absolutely sure.

How did they know?

Women who self-nominated as pre-menopausal were asked if they had thought about menopause. Exactly half had thought about it but their ideas were very vague. Here we have the first indication of a theme that recurs in this book: menopause is not given much consideration until you start experiencing symptoms.

Most of the women (71%) said they were aware of certain signs of menopause. Most of these women associated hot flushes and cessation of menstruation with the onset of menopause. Table 2.2 illustrates what all women surveyed saw as the certain signs of menopause. Of the women surveyed 38% (321) had experienced what they said were certain signs of menopause. Figure 2.1 illustrates the various ways in which these women gauged their menopausal status. As the graph shows, age was the key indicator. This raises the question: at what age do women think midlife begins?

Table 2.2 Certain signs of menopause

Sign	% of total women surveyed
Cessation of menses	33
Hot flushes	33
Tiredness	2
Depression	22
Erratic menses	3
All other signs	7

Midlife women and health status

Thirty-nine per cent of the women who self-nominated as either having experienced or started menopause reported that it began between the ages of 46 and 50, while 25% reported that it started between the ages of 41 and 45.

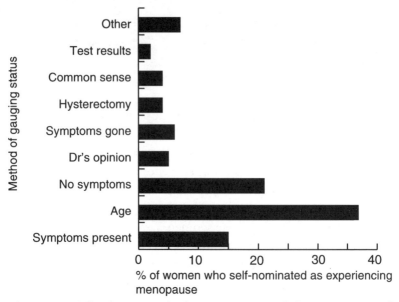

Figure 2.1 The ways in which women gauged their menopausal status.

Women currently being treated for menopause (107) were most likely to be using hormone therapy (84). The next most common category of treatment was vitamins (16), then oil of evening primrose (12). However, 6 women reported being treated with anti-depressants and 2 with psychotherapeutic drugs.

To understand what younger women think about menopause, we asked them if they had thought about it — the majority had not. As previously noted, women who self-nominated as pre-menopausal were evenly divided between those who had thought about it and those who hadn't.

The women in our survey who took HRT for menopause were asked if they expected to continue with the treatment and, if so, for how long. In much of the popular literature HRT is presented as a treatment that provides long-term health benefits through the prevention of cardiovascular disease and osteoporosis. Over half of the women expected to continue taking HRT for the long term. Only 9% of women felt it was a short-term option, 26% were unsure about whether they would continue taking hormone treatment and 7% did not wish to continue. Asked how confident they were about taking the treatment, most were either very confident (37%) or fairly confident (38%); while 17% had mixed feelings and 8% of the women were very unsure. This is the generation of women who probably first used the contraceptive pill and lived through its developments. HRT is at a similar stage to the contraceptive pill in its early days. It has yet to be used by a cohort of women for many years and, as later chapters show, these women were rarely confident of its benefits or safety.

IMAGES OF MENOPAUSE

We brought to the data expectations framed by our own experiences and our knowledge of the popular debate on menopause. These told us that the topic was 'taboo' and that menopause is always viewed in a negative way, with competing dominant images. As chapter 3 shows, these messages come from a range of popular and professional literature. The medicalisation of menopause led to a debate in terms of illness, deterioration and possible 'cure' of hormone deficiency. Out of that debate emerged feminist-led efforts in the popular literature to help women think positively about menopause, these texts portrayed it as a new stage of maturity, wisdom and freedom from the woman's lot of childbearing and nurturing. Both these strands of thought are backed by the assumption that women think about menopause negatively, society picturing the menopausal woman and, later, the ageing woman, as sad, unattractive or sick. Thus when we set out, with the survey, to discover the dominant images, we had every reason to expect they would be powerful and negative.

Menopause has historically been reported in the literature as a taboo subject and a life stage that is viewed in a negative way. To understand how such a history has or has not impacted on different generations of Australian women's images of midlife, we asked women from all age groups to circle words (from a given list) they associated with menopause. The task of asking women about images proved an interesting methodological challenge, as we did not want to imply that women should have an image and offered none. The words selected were those that recurred in the three-year qualitative study. One hundred and sixteen women did not select any word to describe menopause, suggesting they did not have a set image of it. Nevertheless, most of the women had some type of image of menopause. Younger women were more likely to circle words than older women, suggesting that they have stronger preconceived ideas of a life stage they have not yet reached. Following is the question we asked, and the range of words women could choose from for their answer:

> *These are some of the words women have used to describe menopause to us. Please circle the ones that fit your idea of menopause.*
>
> | | | | |
> |---|---|---|---|
> | new stage | no change | tired | empty nest |
> | non-event | wisdom | stigma | new zest |
> | beginning old age | myths | health risk | private |
> | relief | danger | frustrating | avoidable |
> | unattractive | taking stock | taboo | sad |
> | illness | infertility | lonely | freedom |
> | pain | losing sexuality | threat | embarrassing |
> | peace | journey | | |

It was impossible in a mail-out survey to understand how women negotiated which words fitted their ideas of menopause. The same set of words were piloted in some of our taped interviews, however, and these transcripts gave us a chance to hear how women considered each word before selecting which word or words matched their image of menopause. Jane, one of the women we piloted the questionnaire with, reacted in the following way when presented with the task of choosing words that fitted her idea of menopause:

'New stage'. Because I've grown and developed, and I know that it's no major event. 'Non-event', because I'm hoping it will be. Wouldn't it be wonderful if you were one of those who got a period this month, and next month nothing. So, that's why I've circled that. That's with a lot of hope. Why is it going to be a 'relief'? Because I won't have to have a bloody period every . . . once you are at this stage . . . I've had my tubes tied ages ago, so why am I having these things every month. I've had my kids, I really don't . . . I've got to that stage . . . I think that's what happens to a lot of people, 'Oh, my God, no more children.' I went through that. I had to force myself to look at that when I got my tubes tied. So, I don't think I'll do that. What does 'avoidable' mean? It's non-avoidable. I'll put 'non' on top of that. I don't mind the stopping of the periods it's the rest of the stuff. 'Taking stock', no. That's right. 'Sad'. I suppose just a little . . . I started [menstruating] at 16 . . . say if I started [menopause] at 45, that's a hell of a lot of your life that you've been a certain way. So, I suppose it's sad as in . . . Look, I've even done a little circle. Just a little sad. 'Infertility'. Yes, because I still worry, just in case those things come undone. 'Freedom'. Again, freedom from . . . I'm pretty good now. I've settled down. Over the last year, twenty-eight days, I'm going so well. So, freedom from that, because you still wonder, and I get that couple of days of pain and the aching legs. 'Peace'. I think it will be, because there is always that . . . the going through it may not be peace, but the afterwards. Looking at things, I don't think it will be 'embarrassing' going through it unless of course you have hot flushes, and you are standing there talking to somebody and have to explain. Because it is the natural way of things. You could go on forever having babies. If you stayed young . . . no, you need to go through . . . I look at my Mum . . . she's gone through it, and she had a few things . . . hot flushes and things, but she didn't have anything major. Every now and then I think to myself, 'don't try and hurry it'. I have to hold myself back. I look at the two of them. The kids are older, and I think, 'wouldn't it be nice'. Then again, enjoy the stage I'm at now. Don't hurry it. The only changes that I can see myself going through, and this is the only thing I dread about getting older, is losing the kids. I'm one of these silly people . . . I can't stand the thought of them not being here.

The success of this technique seemed evident — until we looked for the dominant images. On first viewing, the data showed no agreement. Menopause seemed image-less! Extraordinarily, despite the confident assertions in popular and professional literature, no words that would indicate the stereotypes were consistently, or even frequently, selected. But then there were no words consistently selected, and no groups of words consistently selected together by all women.

We searched in vain for patterns across the whole sample. None of the words were dominant. Cluster analysis failed to indicate clusters of words being selected together. Retreating to simple viewing of the data, word by word, we pieced together the explanation. There was no overall set of words that grouped across the sample, not because there are no images of menopause, but because they shift and are patterned by age. The graphs of each word by age vividly showed that images appear and fade with different age groups, suggesting they are mediated by life stage and women's experience.

Overall, younger women were more likely to have negative images, while those of older women, post-menopause, were more positive. The younger women were also more likely to circle a greater number of words than older women. Did they have stronger ideas of the words associated with a life stage they had not yet reached, or less fixed ideas? And, most intriguingly, the midlife age groups were the least likely to show clear images, suggesting both confusion and a process of rethinking stereotypes as experience came into play.

Accepted Images

There was no single set of words that could be constructed to present an image that women from all age groups held. The word 'freedom' was the only word that came close to being selected by women of all age groups at a constant level. But the word freedom could mean many things — here we were confronted by the limitations of a survey in which we could not ask women to explain their choice of words. Possible interpretations include many freedoms; the most likely associations of the word freedom in regard to menopause are freedom from child-rearing, the pressures of work, menstruation and worrying about unwanted pregnancies.

A word that would logically fit with freedom was clearly 'relief' but this was selected by very few women, and not by all age groups. If you are granted freedom surely you would feel relieved! Freedom perhaps presents a double-edged sword. It is an attractive prospect to be free from menstruation, working and worrying about unplanned pregnancies but once you are free from these you are reaching your older years. However freedom was not significantly linked with 'beginning old age'. Other possible interpretations for the word freedom include to do or be something else. But freedom did not cluster across the sample with other words suggesting a 'new stage', 'wisdom' or 'journey'.

REJECTED STEREOTYPES

None of the images most assumed in the literature were supported by these women. The sad, unattractive, sexless females often asserted to be society's image of midlife did not feature strongly. Younger women had a more negative image of menopause but it was not extreme. The popular claim that menopause is taboo was clearly contradicted, the word 'taboo' was chosen by less than 10% of the women across all age groups. The frequent assertion that menopausal women bear the wrath of social stigma was even less supported.

Feminist arguments that menopause is popularly associated with deterioration and risk, and that women feel threatened by this life stage, did not appear in this data — very few women circled the negative words that would represent these feelings. Women did not see menopause as a threat or a life stage that they should find embarrassing. Of all the negative images of menopause none rated as low as that of 'danger'. The women did not have images of gloom and doom as presented in some of the feminist literature. The prevalence of the image of the 'empty-nest' syndrome was also challenged, with well under 10% of women in each age group choosing this word.

AGE AND IMAGES OF MENOPAUSE

The image of menopause as a 'non-event' was clearly accepted more by women who had experienced it, and they were much

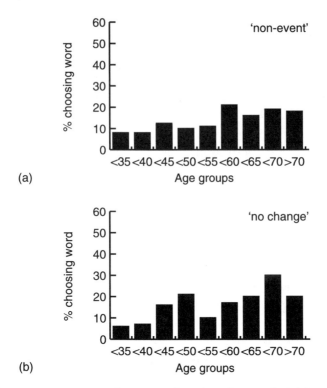

Figure 2.2 Per cent of women choosing the words (a) 'non-event', and (b) 'no change', by age group.

more likely to see menopause as bringing 'no change'. (See Figure 2.2.)

Younger women's images of menopause were more negative than older women's, suggesting that younger women have more reservations about their middle years than those women who are approaching or have gone through them. Acceptance of words associated with the image of dreading menopause ('sad', 'frustrating') decreased with age. Younger women were more likely to ring 'new stage', but this may not have been positive. Younger women were more likely to associate menopause with loss of fertility than older women, this is presumably because childbearing is an issue much more associated with their current life stage. (See Figure 2.3.)

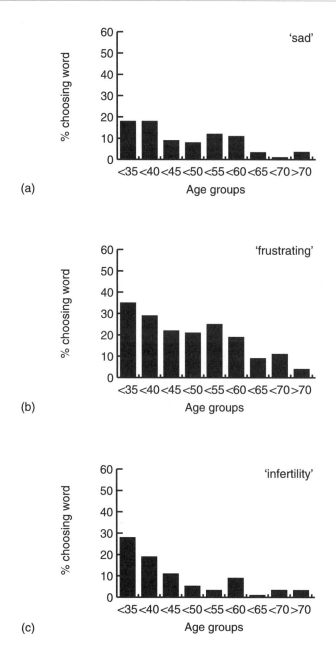

Figure 2.3 Per cent of women choosing the words (a) 'sad', (b) 'frustrating', and (c) 'infertility', by age group.

Menopause as a medical issue

Images of the ill, sick woman did not feature strongly in this survey's results, suggesting that these assumptions need to be rethought. Equally interesting was the absence of the stereotype assumed in much feminist critique of medical authority. Women of all ages showed little acceptance of images of menopause as unavoidable or as illness. 'Health risk', 'illness' and 'pain' were among the least accepted words. But the words suggesting the 'wise woman' image promoted in recent feminist writing — 'wisdom', 'new zest' and 'peace' — were equally unacceptable.

Shifted images

The patterns of words circled seem to show the interplay between limited knowledge and experience. For midlife women, images of menopause faded in importance depending on what they were currently experiencing. The fact that there was no single image for midlife women shows that it is a time of individual growth and change, which reflects women's understanding of their new experiences. These experiences are highly varied, rapidly changing and closely interwoven with other aspects of their lives, especially family change, workforce participation and sexuality.

Are social attitudes changing?

Did women perceive that social attitudes towards menopause and midlife were changing, and if so in what direction? At the end of the survey we asked women, 'What seem to you to be the current social attitudes to menopause?' We offered no suggestions, just space to write a reply. Following this question we asked women, 'Do you think these attitudes are changing?' Interestingly, 212 women did not respond to this question, suggesting that they had no perception of whether there had been any change in society's attitudes. Perhaps they had given up the task of filling out the survey as these were the last questions. But the women who responded wrote pages on this topic, especially older women who wanted to share their experiences of menopause. Often, women wrote in detail of the ways they were treated compared with the ways their daughters have experienced midlife. Over a third of the women surveyed said that they didn't know if society's attitudes had changed. The open-ended responses suggest that these women either were truly unaware of the current social attitudes (a typical response was 'no idea'), or had experienced menopause and did not wish to consider or reflect on what society's attitudes were, as one older woman commented:

> Women of my age group. We are all too busy enjoying life, playing bowls and golf, working for the CWA, Red Cross et cetera, and generally enjoying our freedom from the stresses of rearing children, earning a living . . .

While a narrow majority of women surveyed felt that society's attitudes were changing, only 14% of the women felt that there had been a great change in society's attitudes. Another 38% said that there had been some change. When asked what the changes were, women reported that the topic is now discussed more openly. Typical comments from women included the following:

> Subject talked about a lot more openly and freely than in the past.

> More often open discussion. Not the forbidden subject of latter years — needs to be more of the same.

> Everything is discussed openly about everything, perhaps too much so, like advertising for ladies' pads on TV — is that really necessary? Some things are private.

Women who reported that social attitudes had changed related this to the availability of more information, which provided them with options to deal with menopause. Information was often linked to the availability of medical treatment:

> I'm glad it is a more open society today and people can get help and guidance for menopause, and don't have to feel isolated. It is not taboo to talk about these things today which is great.

> I think the modern women are more well-informed and more women have access to caring medical treatment with Medicare.

> Women are investigating menopause and making informed decisions

on hormone replacement therapy and other ways of coping. Most of my friends have a very positive attitude.

Great changes and more acceptance across the community. Definitely much more help and information available to women. Clinics are more widespread GPs are learning more to help women instead of [referring them] to a specialist.

Women linked changing social attitudes with a general increase in the interest in women's health issues and their social status:

> Accepting Women's health needs as important, giving them attention. Listening to women and their health problems. Preparing women for the different health stages in their life.

> Doctors are more understanding of the problems women face during this period. And [better at] recognising the symptoms at [an] early stage, therefore ensuring women receive the proper advice and treatment.

Women who felt that there had been some change (38%) in society's attitudes towards menopause had similar reasons for reaching this conclusion as the women who reported that there had been great changes: namely that information was more widely available and that the topic was discussed. Some women also suggested that the change in societal attitudes was related to women accepting the changes themselves:

> More publicity. Women [are] more prepared to speak publicly on [the] issue. This may be confined to middle-class women. However, I feel people are more aware and accepting of menopause as a 'real' condition, physically and mentally.

> Like many other women of my generation, any mention of menopause was 'unladylike', now openness is a necessary part of living.

> Slow movement towards women taking charge of their own bodily and emotional experiences. Everyone I know accepts the changes that may affect them, and tries to take them in their stride and seek medical advice.

> People are more willing to discuss their symptoms and accept the fact that there are changes occurring in their body, and their lives.

Interestingly, even though 16% of women said that they felt there had been little or no change, many mentioned changes in their comments. Perhaps they did not perceive that these small changes represented any real change:

> None of my friends or family are going through this stage — [I] don't really know enough to comment. The only thing I have noticed is that women seem to talk more freely about menopause (as with discussing periods). It's not a taboo subject anymore.

Conclusion

This data has revealed that women's images of menopause are not negative and that women see social attitudes as changing. The process of constructing an image or set of images about menopause can perhaps be likened to an orchestral performance, with different instruments and melodies playing at different times — fading and intensifying as one element takes over another. The women in our survey certainly recognised images of menopause, but they were by no means uniform.

There is no evidence for the usual stereotypes of menopause as a taboo subject, a period of illness, a 'curable disease', or for the 'wise women' images of feminist writing. So much for the stereotypes! This book is about the ways in which women construct their understandings and how these shift in the interplay between women's knowledge and experience. Understanding menopause is a process and women are agents in this process.

Very little has been written about the ways women at midlife access information about menopause and what types of information are available to them. We were interested to compare the information available in the popular literature with what women reported accessing. The following chapter details our findings through a review of the popular literature and an analysis of the material the women said they accessed.

3
MIRRORS OF MENOPAUSE — THE POPULAR LITERATURE

Carmel Seibold and Nicole Davis

Women experiencing menopause in the late twentieth century are not facing a situation where menopause is shrouded in mystery and half truths. Our survey showed that, contrary to some critiques, menopause is not seen as taboo.[1] Nor is there a lack of information on the subject — the amount of attention menopause has received in the last few years heralds a change from menopause as women's business to menopause as everyone's business!

Unlike their mothers, women now have many sources of information outside the medical system. Medical knowledge as defined by doctors is the subject of subsequent chapters. Here, we look at the primary sources of popular information, magazines and books. What messages did they convey to women and what was their potential for influencing experience?

The women in the survey and the women interviewed support the findings of several studies and what is expressed in the popular literature, that women often do not give menopause a thought until they are menopausal (Beyenne 1986; Greer 1991; Sheehy 1993). Once they experience symptoms the ways in which they seek information vary depending on the availability of resources and their awareness of what information can be accessed. Our survey suggests that the popular media, including women's magazines, feature strongly as a source of information about menopause. We asked women in the survey to select from a list their sources of information on menopause. Over a third (38%) circled 'magazines, TV or newspapers'. 'Doctor' came second (28%), only just beating 'mother' (27%), and 'books' and 'friends' came next (both 26%). Trailing behind were 'pamphlets' (18%) and 'other family members' (12%), with 'other health professional' scoring a mere 5%. It is worth noting, however, that the survey included women who were pre-menopausal.

MAGAZINES AS A SOURCE OF INFORMATION

The popularity of magazines among the women in our studies is not surprising. Australians spend $790 million on consumer magazines a year, making them the largest readers of magazines in the world per capita. On average each Australian reads sixteen magazines a year (*Magazines 2000* 1996). A typical response to questions on sources of information about menopause was: 'Oh magazines, you know I read [them] . . . and any articles I can find.'

Not all women saw articles in magazines as expressing the definitive opinion. Women who were educated in the health field checked their advice. One woman, a nurse, had this to say: 'I do tend to pick up magazines in dentists and places like that and if they have an article I'm interested in, say on menopause, I read it — but then I like to check its sources.' Others questioned whether the information provided was balanced: 'There is not a lot of information around that is easily obtainable. And a lot of what is written is very biased opinion.'

The data suggest magazine articles on midlife and menopause were influential in several ways. For women not actively seeking information, reading magazines triggered self-reflection about women and menopause: '[Magazines] probably started me thinking about things. I'm a bit more understanding about what other people are going through. The only chance I get to read anything is in a magazine . . .' They could also operate as a means of clarification: 'I tend to read an article in a magazine and it helps clarify something I've heard or the doctor's said.' Magazine articles also provided a basis for discussion among women about issues relevant to midlife.

So what messages did women pick up from the magazines? Amanda Jenkins reviewed four popular Australian magazines for our project for the period 1986 to 1992: the *Australian Women's Weekly, Family Circle, Ita* and *New Woman*.[2] The message in these magazines is predominantly one of support for HRT, with the associated emphasis on menopause as a deficiency disease with significant consequences if left untreated. In a large proportion of the articles HRT is stressed as a means of preventing osteoporosis. As Sandra Coney (1993) has noted the spectre of the dowager's hump is present, even in the relatively well-balanced articles, causing women who don't experience problems to rethink their approach to menopause as a natural event. For example McKenzie (1986), acknowledging that her description of risk factors for osteoporosis (which are extensive) sounds grim, states 'until recently all women could expect to suffer some disability from osteoporosis [authorities generally agree between one-third and one-quarter are at risk] if they lived beyond the age of 65. Women born since 1940 need have no fear of this bone disorder. If we heed the advice abundantly available, we can take steps to prevent it.' The advice, in a nutshell, is exercise, dietary calcium and HRT.

Other articles take a more even-handed approach. An 'Update on osteoporosis' (1989) opens with 'There are simple measures you can take to prevent this crippling disease.' The emphasis is on a calcium-rich diet as well as exercise and HRT. The authority cited is a dietitian. The side-effects of HRT are mentioned along with the benefits and the assurance that it is a very common and effective treatment that has been around for ten years. Women are urged to be proactive in having HRT prescribed by their general practitioners if they see it as beneficial, 'as not all GPs are up to date in the management of menopause'.

In the late 1980s and early 1990s there was increasing interest in HRT because of the protection it offers against cardiovascular disease and osteoporosis (Cabot, Wilson & Garratt 1989; Edison 1988; Weissen 1991). Professor Barry Wren of the Centre for Management of Menopause in Sydney (noted by Edison [1988] to be 'an international authority on post menopausal women'), recommends HRT for the majority of menopausal women, even in some cases for those with oestrogen-dependent cancers. While he does take a whole-person approach, in terms of recognising other stressors that may impinge on midlife women, his focus is biomedical, describing menopause as 'a complex medical problem requiring education, counselling and supportive therapy'. He likens menopause to diabetes placing it firmly in the category of a deficiency disease and recommends HRT. At the same time, although viewing women largely in terms of traditional roles, he does note that women at midlife are experiencing children leaving home, loss of reproductive potential and elderly and ill parents. Although he considers that these factors have nothing to do with oestrogen deficiency, at the same time he seems to be saying HRT can do a lot for you, and what it can't do counselling and education, presumably from a medical source, can.

In all this material there is a heavy emphasis on the voice of medical authority. In some cases the articles or health reports are written or co-written by a doctor or menopause researcher (Cabot 1989; Cabot, Wilson & Garratt 1989; McKenzie 1986, 1990). In a number of other articles a doctor, either associated with a menopause clinic or an acknowledged authority, is cited and quoted uncritically. (Beasley 1989; Edison 1988; Hershon 1991; Kennedy 1990; Powell 1991; Turner 1990). For example, Professor Burger is cited by Powell (1991) as stating:

> Every woman at the time of menopause should have the opportunity to be assessed and counselled about the appropriate way to manage things. She should know what the options, risks and benefits are and then make her decision. And judging by the evidence that is not a difficult decision to make.

However the biomedical perspective is varied even in these simple presentations. Not all the articles on HRT stressed menopause as a deficiency disease. Some only refer to HRT for the relief of symptoms:

> Finally as we women of a certain age know, the BIG M, menopause has had a bad press. New and safer methods of oestrogen replacement have freed many women from the hot flushes and decreased vaginal lubrication commonly associated with the cessation of menstruation. (Cohen 1991)

Although the majority of articles in popular magazines favoured HRT, particularly if citing medical experts, there were those that also addressed the health risks associated with HRT (Kerr 1990), along with those that presented information about menopause and recommended natural management such as diet, calcium and vitamin supplements and exercise (Kennedy 1990). An alternative view was provided by an article titled 'Osteoporosis the unnecessary disease', which appeared in *Ita*, a magazine whose articles in this period showed a definite bias towards HRT. It was written by Dr Vic Barker (1990), who practises in New Zealand and purports to treat osteoporosis successfully without surgery or drugs. His emphasis is on diet, exercise and attention to posture. He also notes his difficulty in having papers accepted at medical conferences covering osteoporosis. A few articles treat midlife solely as a life stage — a time of transition and a rite of passage (Armstrong 1990), but these offer a different imbalance and, as Amanda Jenkins notes, do not acknowledge 'that midlife may bring physiological as well as psychological changes'.

A cursory look at more recent editions of the four magazines reviewed showed that there was a dearth of material dealing with menopause from a medical perspective. What is starting to appear are articles with a clear bias towards alternative methods of treatment, such as herbal remedies. For example, the *Australian Women's Weekly* (September 1994) published an excerpt from a book advocating alternative therapies.

The overall emphasis, with regard to menopause, in the four popular magazines is on self-care, stressing the importance of diet, exercise and healthy living along with HRT. The general impression given in the majority of articles published in the late

1980s and early 1990s is that if women ignore the advice of the medical profession regarding prevention of disease through HRT they are not taking responsibility for their health. An article by Bunty Turner (1990), states:

> If more women looked after themselves properly they would stop placing their health in so much risk. Not enough have regular check-ups. Not enough have mammography to check for breast cancer. And certainly far too few women have the good news that osteoporosis can be diagnosed, treated and prevented.

Another message for midlife women that relates to self-care comes from articles dealing with maintaining a youthful and attractive appearance in midlife. The role models are exotic: Joan Collins, Raquel Welch, Elizabeth Taylor 'and our own Maggie Tabberer and Sonia McMahon' (*Australian Women's Weekly*, March 1988): and in *Ita* (Lord 1989), Coco Chanel and Jackie Onassis are cited. They are to be emulated by taking care of your appearance and not letting yourself go. Midlife women are not permitted the luxury of sinking into the middle-aged spread without guilt. Plastic surgery is another option for the midlife woman — perpetuating the beauty myth into middle age (Armstrong 1990; Beaumont 1990). In the period under review only *New Woman* published articles that challenged the beauty myth (Gross 1991; Pogrebin 1989). Gross cautions against buying into the youth equals beauty myth and is critical of ageism and age shame. Pogrebin, in a somewhat humorous vein and in line with Greer's (1991) thesis, challenges the myth replacing the myth of ageism, namely that women are now successfully growing older with pride and affirmation. She says she hasn't quite been able to pull it off yet, but to ask her again in a year — when she's 51.

WOMEN AND MENOPAUSE TEXTS

The women we talked with sometimes read popular texts as well as magazines. But in all our data only four authors' texts were referred to by name: Sandra Cabot (*Menopause: You Can Give It a Miss!*, 1991), Germaine Greer (*The Change: Women, Ageing and the Menopause*, 1991), Derek Llewellyn-Jones (several books) and Linda Ojeda (*Menopause without Medicine*, 1989). The first three authors are Australian and both Cabot and Greer were heavily marketed at the time of the studies (1992–93).

Reading of popular texts on menopause usually occurred once a woman was menopausal, or in a few cases when same-age friends were experiencing menopause. Magazine articles often directed women to particular books, which were then frequently shared among a group of friends:

> I think I saw an article in a magazine about this particular book and then a friend mentioned it, she had borrowed it from someone else and it was a good one . . . It is written by a woman going through the menopause at the time. God it was funny, I can't remember, there were a few little books around all at the same time.

Another woman suggests a link between reading magazines and then seeking out popular texts:

> Just by reading in magazines. I did buy a book about menopause . . . It interests me mainly because I've got friends going through it. So, it's really what I just learn from reading.

Reference texts were also recommended by health professionals at menopause information nights and workshops.[3] Greer's book *The Change* tended to feature heavily among recommended references in 1991 and 1992. A community-health nurse told us: 'The Community Health Centre has bought Germaine Greer's new book *The Change* and it will be available to be borrowed soon when some of the staff have read it.'

Books were used as a source of both information and reassurance:

> Why, I thought yes they say it is menopause. But until you actually read it and you see it there in black and white do you fully understand? Because you may have an aching muscle, you may have tender breasts, and you think what the hell is happening — is it to you only? The only information that you're getting is what other people tell you until you actually get it yourself and read it — you know, you can say, this is why I am getting this, this is why I am feeling like it . . .

The well-known Llewellyn-Jones book, *Everywoman: A Gynaecological Guide to Life* (1989), was also noted as a reference. Several women referred to this book as a general resource and one woman noted that she had had it on her shelves for a number of years. Another woman, in reference to the book by Llewellyn-Jones and Abraham (*Menopause*, 1988), said:

> [In] the Derek Llwellyn-Jones book I found the first probably two chapters useful where it was very general . . . and probably only talked about symptoms and how the age range can range from thirties to fifties or whatever. Once they got a bit technical I found it boring . . . I couldn't be bothered reading it.

The Change featured in many of the interviews. Responses to it varied widely. One interviewee used it as a source of information and reassurance:

> Germaine's book *The Change* sits on my pillow. I went to school with her and think her book is well researched. When I used to wake up in the middle of the night thinking I was dying I would grab her book, look up the relevant section via the index, and go back to sleep reassured.

Another was singularly unimpressed: 'A friend gave me Germaine's book. It's the most depressing thing I've ever read. I rang her up and said "get it out of here".'

APPROACHES TO MENOPAUSE IN POPULAR TEXTS

Popular texts tend to be more varied in their approach to menopause than magazines and a significant number do not favour HRT. A number of popular texts, whether or not they advocate HRT, provide enough information about it to enable women to make up their own minds. Freya Hedlam and Carmel Seibold reviewed a representative sample of popular texts covering the late 1980s and early 1990s. They could be said to fall into three broad groups: those with a biomedical slant that favour HRT (Beard & Curtis 1988; Bromwich 1989; Cabot 1991; Coope 1984; Hailes 1986; Kearsley 1990); those that attempt to give a balanced view (Ballinger & Walker 1987; Bennett & Degeling 1988; Dickson &

Henriques 1988; Greenwood 1989; Hunter 1990; Llewellyn-Jones & Abraham 1988; Shreeve 1986); and those advocating 'menopause naturally' (Doress & Siegal 1987; Greer 1991; Ojeda 1989; Reitz 1987). Regardless of their stance a number of texts include information beyond the physical symptoms and talk about menopause as transition (Greenwood 1984; Hunter 1990). Some, more philosophical in nature, like Greer's, wax lyrical about menopause as transition and a rite of passage.

The most well-known Australian text arguing the case for HRT is Sandra Cabot's *Menopause: You Can Give It a Miss!*, Whereas authors of popular texts with a medical bias written in the 1960s emphasised HRT as a means of relieving symptoms and remaining 'feminine forever' (Wilson 1966), the current emphasis as reflected in Cabot's book is on HRT as protection against osteoporosis and cardiovascular disease; relief of symptoms associated with menopause, while still important, is a secondary consideration. Cabot also recommends the use of alternative treatments or complementary therapies, often advocated along with HRT.

Llewellyn-Jones and Abraham's *Menopause*, as an example of a book claiming to provide a balanced view, states that the authors set out to inform readers without patronising them, and they generally achieve this aim, citing studies that provide evidence for and against various viewpoints such as calcium supplements for the prevention of bone loss post-menopause. But the balance of the book is presented within the medical context. The text is scientific and technical and takes an essentially medical view of menopause. The approach, while informing and allowing the individual woman to make up her mind, tends to give the impression of favouring HRT. Shreeve's *Overcoming the Menopause Naturally* (1986), on the other hand, quite clearly sees menopause as a natural event in a woman's development and takes account of the psychic and emotional aspects of menopause. At the same time she addresses the question of HRT in a balanced fashion and while not actively promoting it neither does she come across as anti-HRT.

Among the books advocating natural interpretations of menopause and alternative treatments, Germaine Greer's *The Change* includes a comprehensive discussion of both HRT and alternative therapies. She is generally opposed to HRT, but is also cautious in her approach to the use of various alternative therapies. While advocating non-invasive therapies such as yoga and transcendental meditation, she warns against the wholehearted adoption of alternative therapies for managing menopause on the basis that research as to the efficacy of herbs, for example, is scanty.[4]

Texts that advocate experiencing menopause naturally and those that aim to provide a balanced approach often make reference to the multiple stresses women at menopause are exposed to (Dickson & Henriques 1988, p. 34). In the case of a feminist analysis these symptoms will be put down to a sense of entrapment in the female role, 'a sense of being "gypped"' and a need for empowerment in midlife (Greer 1991, p. 113). Texts with a medical bias also make reference to psychosocial stresses that may be occurring at midlife. However Cabot, after recommending 'some self nurturing' such as 'a holiday, a regular massage or t'ai chi', moves straight on to 'the long term effects of oestrogen deficiency' (1991, p. 26).

Greer also stresses the pervasiveness of the images of menopausal women as potentially 'crazy' which still persist in the 1990s. She traces the historical construction of this image from the clinical psychiatry lectures of Kraepelin in France in the 1800s, and texts such as J. M. Fothergill's, *The Maintenance of Health*, published in England in 1874, which contended that the asylums, the graveyards and the divorce courts were full of women for whom the change of life had caused severe strain (Fothergill, cited in Greer 1991, p. 96). Greer itemises a number of publications that challenged Fothergill's contention, including *A Manual of Psychological Medicine* by John Charles Bucknill and Daniel H. Tuke. Bucknill and Tuke, reviewing the same study on which Fothergill had based his conclusions, found that of 1720 women admitted to Bethlem Asylum 'change of life' was the least common cause of insanity (Buchnill & Tuke, p. 260, cited in Greer 1991, p. 98). Greer laments the pervasiveness of this image, even to this day, for two reasons: because it makes midlife women fearful of madness accompanying the menopause and, just as importantly, because it does not permit midlife women the luxury of depression and rage. Greer feels that depression might more correctly be considered misery and that it 'comes from without and within' (1991, p. 268). She sees the primary cause of this misery as the stigma attached to ageing women and considers rage may be justifiable given the situation of many midlife women.

An example of the pervasiveness of this outmoded medical representation of menopausal women can be found in the disturbing introductory paragraph to Sandra Cabot's popular text:

> An imbalance or lack of hormones can shatter your life. Hormones are vital to make you sexually responsive, passionate, sensitive and to sustain mental drive. According to consultant gynaecologist John Studd of the Menopause clinic at King's College Hospital, London, adequate amounts of female sex hormones keep women 'out of the orthopaedic wards, the divorce courts and the madhouse'. Before Hormone Replacement Therapy (HRT) became available, a significant percentage of menopausal women suffered a severe midlife crisis which was called in medical terminology 'involutional melancholia'. This old-fashioned term [note only the term, not the sentiments, is considered old-fashioned] describes the total shrinking of the mind and the body that could occur without the presence of the sex hormones. Some of these women became so profoundly depressed that they were institutionalised for the rest of their lives. (1991, p. 15)

The refutation of the sentiments expressed in these opening paragraphs can be found in research studies carried out from the 1950s through to the 1980s. These studies found that medical opinion of midlife menopausal women as depressed, withdrawn and crazy was based on research carried out on women hospitalised with depression, or attending clinics (Bart & Grossman 1978; Donovan 1951; Polit & LaRocco 1980). The assumptions on which the original notions were founded had, as Greer noted, a historical base.

Clearly the HRT debate overshadows the popular texts as well as the magazines. It is possible to identify two major models represented in both sources of women's reading, the biomedical model and the alternative health model. The term 'alternative health model' is preferred to 'natural model' as it includes those articles and books that advocate herbal remedies and alternative approaches to viewing and managing menopause. For example, Reitz's book *Menopause a Positive Approach* (1987) takes a comprehensive view of overall health management in menopause and stresses nutrition supplements, exercise and a positive selfimage. It is feminist in orientation and clearly anti-HRT. The majority of popular texts regardless of which model they favour advocate a healthy lifestyle, stress the importance of limiting one's intake of alcohol and caffeine, promote exercise in moderation, and acknowledge the problems of midlife women such as care of elderly parents and coping with teenage children. Most modern texts favouring the so-called 'biomedical model' also draw on alternative (or complementary) approaches to managing menopause. The essential differences appear to be their favouring the widespread prescription of HRT and the manner in which they conceptualise certain beliefs about menopause.

Not all popular texts advocating an alternative to the biomedical model of menopause clearly identify a philosophical position. An exception is Greer's *The Change*. In terms of popular literature it could be said, along with Sandra Coney's book *The Menopause Industry* (1993), to have taken the challenge to the biomedical model out of academia and into the popular arena.

BACKGROUND TO THE DEBATE
THE BIOMEDICAL MODEL

The biomedical model in a purist sense was hard to find in the popular literature. However it has certainly dominated the recent debates on menopause. Bell (1987) and Coney (1993) chronicle the history of the medicalisation of women's bodies from the nineteeth century to the present day. Bell (1987) notes that with the advent of the medical specialty of endocrinology in the 1930s menopause was identified as a deficiency disease. The development of hormonal therapies further established this concept. Initially oestrogen replacement therapy was prescribed as a means of relieving symptoms and remaining 'feminine forever' (Wilson 1966). Studies in the mid-1970s demonstrating an association between oestrogen and uterine cancer (Smith et al. 1975; Zeil & Finkle 1975) saw a more conservative approach to prescription of oestrogen being adopted. The addition of progesterone to HRT, shown to protect against endometrial cancer (Gambrell 1986), and several timely studies confirming HRT as effective in retarding bone loss (Ettinger et al. 1985; Riggs & Melton 1986) saw a return to widespread prescription of it. Research was also emerging that showed that oestrogen decreased the risk of women suffering from cardiovasular diseases, such as heart attacks and strokes (Ross et al. 1987). The emergence of these studies, particularly those demonstrating a link between HRT and prevention of osteoporosis, saw women's magazines being targeted by pharmaceutical companies as a means of marketing HRT to midlife women (Coney 1993). The emphasis on the biomedical model in articles on menopause in women's magazines dates from the mid-1980s. Bell (1987) has noted that four players were instrumental in the marketing of HRT: scientists, medical doctors, drug companies and the state.

THE ALTERNATIVE HEALTH MODEL

The alternative health model tends to draw on a range of literature, most of it in the critical feminist category, to support the view that menopause is a natural event (Dickson 1990; Guillemin 1994; McCrea 1983; McPherson 1981, 1985, 1992). Francis McCrea, one of the leaders of the women's health movement of the early 1970s, viewed the treatment of menopause with oestrogen therapy 'as exploitation of women and an insidious form of social control' (1983, p. 111). McCrea also considered that the scientific and medical view of menopause individualised the problems of menopausal women and by so doing succeeded in averting accountability from the social structures that assign women to a maligned and precarious status in our culture. An alternative view of women's health grew out of the feminist movement and the formation of such organisations as the Boston Women's Health Collective. The publication of *Our Bodies Ourselves* in 1976 emphasised self-care and women taking control of their bodies. The approach to menopause stressed the need to identify the stereotypes attached to women ageing in a 'white male dominated culture [that] devalues ageing and being old, especially where women are concerned' (Phillips & Rakusen 1985, p. 446). Another body of work that challenged the stereotypes was cross-cultural research, which demonstrated that wherever there is a rise in status in midlife there is a consequent lack of symptoms and pathology associated with menopause (Beyenne 1986; Datan 1986; Davis 1986).

A number of books now being read are set in the context of valuing women's experiences and representing menopause as transition and as a rite of passage (Downing 1991; Greer 1991; Mankovitz 1984; Taylor & Coverdale Sumrall 1991). These texts continue to challenge the stereotypes and provide an alternative view. As well as challenging the stereotypes the alternative health model advocates a natural approach to dealing with menopause recommending a healthy lifestyle, limiting one's intake of caffeine and alcohol, regular exercise and vitamin and calcium supplements. More recently so-called natural approaches to managing menopause, such as yoga, meditation and herbs, have been included in the range of options suggested.

There is no doubt the critical feminist writings and studies of menopause (Dickson 1990; McCrea 1983; McPherson 1981, 1985) have influenced current popular writings. The identification of the medicalisation of women's health *per se*, and menopause in particular, as a form of social control, led to a shift in the understanding of menopause as a medical entity as a social construct. More recent studies (Guillemin 1994) have highlighted the pervasiveness of the medical approach in the management of menopause and the ways in which women, as consumers of the services of menopause clinics, participate in the construction of menopause as a deficiency disease. At the same time she found evidence from interviews with women of a tension between the medical approach of the clinics and the experiences of the women. Alternative approaches and perspectives on menopause offer women other options. This provides women with a seeming range of choices. A number of women in the studies have expressed their confusion at being exposed to a range of options (usually by the general practitioner) and then being asked to choose — usually for or against HRT. This can result, depending on how the options are presented, in no choice at all. However women in the studies do not come across as helpless dupes and a dogmatic approach from either end of the spectrum does not appear helpful. Rather, open debate regarding the range of options available to women along with an accurate representation of the state of research would appear most helpful. One recent Australian text that presents a range of options and the current state of research into HRT is *In Transition a Guide to Menopause* by Dr Deborah Saltman (1994). She states in the final chapter, 'Dealing with uncertainty':

> It is clear that there is a strong body of medical support for the belief that all women should be on hormone replacement therapy. However with many decades of hormone replacement therapy behind us, the picture of menopause as a hormone deficiency disorder is too simplistic. There is mounting evidence that the decision to commence a woman on hormone replacement therapy is hazardous. Several dilemmas are unresolved. First, the cancer risk. For example the risk of cancer of the uterus and the breast have not been eliminated. Second the benefits of hormone replacement therapy have not been balanced against the risks. For example the addition of progesterone to protect the uterus from cancer may defeat the protective effect that oestrogen has on the heart and vessels. Finally a clear-cut long term strategy is still missing, for once on hormone replacement therapy there are no clear cut indicators as to when this treatment should cease. (pp. 146–7)[5]

HOW WOMEN USED INFORMATION FROM MAGAZINES AND POPULAR TEXTS

The survey did not ask specific questions as to how women used information or what caused them to lean towards a particular model or approach to the management of menopause. It would seem true to say, however, that no one, including the authors of the articles or books, can evaluate their impact.

The interviews allowed for a little more scope. In the main women tended, if experiencing distressing symptoms, to seek help from the general practitioner. Prescription of HRT for the relief of symptoms meant that initially the information that was accessed about management of menopause had a heavy biomedical slant, often drawn from pamphlets. For many women for whom HRT had provided significant benefit, any further reading referred to tended to be texts that were pro-HRT or provided a balanced approach.

Alternative approaches were often explored when there was a sense of unease experienced with ongoing use of HRT. It was difficult to ascertain which came first, exposure to the alternative approach, or unease with continued use of HRT. It was probably a combination of the two. Texts advocating alternative models of managing menopause were then the basis for justifying decisions taken. Anne's decision to cease HRT, as noted in chapter 4, was a combination of personal experience and reading Ojeda about alternative methods of managing menopause.

The popular literature presents powerful images of midlife and menopause. It therefore provides a background against which women's experiences can be interpreted within the context of social and cultural discourse. The following chapters explore established images of midlife and menopause and acknowledge the impact of societal and cultural discourse on women's experiences.

4
THE BODY IN MIDLIFE

Carmel Seibold

> The body has been made so problematic for women it is easier to shrug it off and travel as a disembodied spirit. (Rich 1977, p. 40)

In seeking to discover the way a group of single (as in divorced, separated or never married) midlife women reflected on their experiences, including their experiences of midlife and menopause, I found this quote became a refrain.

THE STUDY IN CONTEXT

In 1992 as a divorced, midlife woman, a nurse and a sociologist my interest was in exploring single women's perceptions of midlife and menopause as part of my studies for a PhD. Single women, as in those without partners, appeared to be a group largely ignored in the menopause literature and, given that they comprised one-fifth of the population of women between the ages of 40 and 54 (Australian Bureau of Statistics 1993), they appeared worthy of study. I knew my own experience, while similar to that of my partnered friends, was also qualitatively different. I set forth with a combination of enthusiasm and trepidation and started a midlife saga that has continued to the present day.

I interviewed 20 single midlife women (10 single women and 10 previously married women) twice each, with a twelve-month gap between interviews. In the interim 16 of the women kept diaries. Four women were unable to sustain the discipline of keeping a diary for twelve months. The diaries were a wonderful source of material with one exceeding 15 000 words. An abridged version of this diary appears as chapter 6. Ten women were divorced or separated and 10 women had never married. Fifteen of the women had backgrounds in teaching or nursing, one was a librarian, one a former hairdresser now a university student, one taught music in her home, one had been a home-maker and now had a part-time job in sales, and one had just been made redundant from a position in the service industry. Four of the women, all with backgrounds in teaching, were nuns. I am grateful to all the women for sharing their time and stories with me.

THE BODY AS PROBLEMATIC

A significant theme to emerge from the interviews was the often uneasy relationship women had with their bodies. It became apparent in preliminary analysis of the interviews that the relationship the women had with their bodies prior to midlife affected their response to and management of the midlife and menopausal body. While this may seem self-evident, there is a tendency in viewing the midlife and menopausal body to assume that the relationship women had with their bodies prior to midlife was unproblematic, and that the experience of midlife and menopause occurs in isolation from a pre-midlife and post-menopausal body. Contrary to this assumption I was surprised to find how much time many of the women devoted to describing what I termed the pre-menopausal/pre-midlife body. This despite the fact that although open-ended interviews were used, which allowed the women to explore various aspects of their experiences as midlife women, no specific questions were asked reflecting on their experiences prior to midlife and menopause.

A theme that emerged in many of the interviews was the degree of reflection on the pre-menopausal body undertaken by many of the women. Their experiences of their body prior to midlife and in midlife appeared to be mediated by social expectations and discourse.[1] For me as a feminist researcher this brought to mind Henrietta Moore's (1994) contention that the task for feminist researchers with regard to gender and the body is to work out what bearing social and cultural discourses have on individual experience. Consequently this chapter discusses four sub-themes within the context of the overall theme of the body: working the body, controlling the body, listening to the body, viewing the body; and in conclusion reflects on social and cultural influences on individual experience including the mind–body divide.

WORKING THE BODY

Making the body work was a strong theme. For some women it preceded menopause. Women reflecting on the past recalled ignoring painful menstrual symptoms and coping with potentially embarrassing situations relating to heavy periods. Women in the workforce experienced a menopausal body out of control and spoke of a need to manage the body in order to be competent in the world of work.

Some women used language that suggested that they related to their bodies as objects. The emphasis is on the body as a machine. There is a strong need to control the body and make 'it' work, Alice said:

> It worked for me and I demanded it to work . . . I got the flu every year when I was teaching. Once I stopped teaching I didn't get the flu again and it was a couple of years later I realised that I hadn't got the flu. It was through that welfare work and course of study [Master of Pastoral Care] that I came across this notion — it was like a revelation and I thought 'so that's what that was, I wanted out'. I remember being so relieved once when I had the flu, 'great three weeks off' . . . what I was actually doing to my body didn't come in. It didn't matter what I was feeling, what time of the month it had to perform.

Heavy periods and painful symptoms were kept in the private realm until such time as the risk of not doing something impinged on the public role (Alice again):

Yes, well I never knew if it was normal or not, what I was having, and other women didn't talk about it. Oh god it was painful . . . I had to go home and change my clothes and all that sort of thing . . . What finally got me to the doctor was when I was in a woman's home [visiting in the role of parish assistant] . . . and she had me sitting in her lounge room on a white velvet lounge suite — that's when I decided it was time to go [to the doctor].

Alice acknowledged that within the Catholic tradition, and particularly as a nun, 'we were encouraged to deny our bodies'.

Georgie also recalled the heavy demands placed on her body through long hours and demanding work. The realisation of a greater need to get in touch with her body and seek more time out came as a result of a complete physical breakdown:

GEORGIE: I experienced a real burn-out when I was 38. I had been moved from one school to another, a whole new ministry and a new secondary school. I sort of started the year all right but had no idea that my whole physical health had broken down and then I collapsed and was paralysed for a couple of months.

CARMEL: Did you learn anything from this?

GEORGIE: Yes, I learnt to take time out for myself because on the enneogram [a test identifying personality type] I'm a 2 and and a 2 is mother's little helper. A 2 tries to help out with everybody and meets other people's needs and not your own. So that was really the turning point in my life.

Awareness of the body and 'making it work for you' came at different stages for women in different situations. Some who had children seemed to have more positive experiences of periods, which Joanne described as 'the cycling aspect of my body'. Both periods and pregnancy were often described positively. 'I loved my periods,' Rebecca said, 'I loved being pregnant.'

Awareness of the body at a physical level was intermittent and largely suppressed by single (never married) pre-menopausal women. With the onset of distressing symptoms all those having a natural menopause spoke of a heightened awareness of the body and an inability to ignore the body. This was expressed in relation to menopausal symptoms, such as frequent hot flushes, as a 'body out of control' and with a 'mind of its own'. The body not working adequately was invariably a problem for women in positions of authority and in the public eye. Jane, a senior nurse administrator, on first being interviewed reported:

> Oh, it's been going on for a couple of months now, but it's got worse the last few weeks. I suppose the last month it's been worse. And, at night time, when I'm walking around the wards, the perspiration is just running off me literally. It's like you have just been in the shower and you have got all this perspiration pouring down your face. And they wonder just what's wrong with you. I mean, you feel an absolute drip . . .

Anne speaks of the distress she experienced when hot flushes first occurred and how the associated mental and physical problems built up:

> [Hot flushes] are the most uncomfortable things I have ever lived through, because you are just suddenly hot all over . . . and you feel as though you are almost about to explode. And you are sort of undoing blouses, taking off clothes, opening windows . . . The middle of the night you would wake up, and you would have to fling back the bed-clothes, you would be just boiling hot all of a sudden. And that was extremely uncomfortable . . . probably you could live with the hot flushes and the sweats if you got enough sleep . . . about the same time I started to feel extremely tired . . . I mean you feel tired if you have been busy, or expect it, but I was exhausted, absolutely wrung out. Morning as well as night. You wake up exhausted. I had a lot of headaches, and [became] extremely anxious. I got the palpitations for no reason, and I had this tense anxiety feeling . . .

The body out of control involved mind and memory out of control and again workforce participation was a significant factor. Emotional lability and loss of memory were feared in this context. Menopausal symptoms and the domino effect of lack of sleep and tiredness combined with increasing stress at work impacted on a number of women. Anne, a nurse educator, reflecting back on a period of change at her workplace recalled:

> I completely lost confidence in myself. Probably didn't associate it with menopause for a start because a lot of things were happening with the job. But looking back I think I could have handled it better if I hadn't been menopausal at the same time.

A sense of not being in control physically was part of this lack of confidence:

> There was a real feeling that you had suddenly . . . almost like you were a puppet and someone else was pulling the strings literally. And you didn't have the strength or ability to suddenly grab hold of it and say 'it's my life I'll do with it what I want to do'. And so you really felt that there was someone else taking over your life, you were sort of flying blind . . .

Emotional lability had a significant effect for four women. Anne and Karla saw this as negative because it had the potential to contribute to a less than competent image. Della and Georgie dealt with it quite differently. Georgie saw her emotional response to the students who came to her for counselling as a means of expressing greater empathy. Della as a chaplain had no trouble building it into her work and she perceived this as allowing her space to deal with her emotions:

> CARMEL: Do you find you're more emotional?
> DELLA: Oh yes but in my job to have a good cry isn't such a bad thing. I mean does it matter if I cry easily for two or three days. I mean if I cry here people just think I'm crying for them and they think that is fabulous and it doesn't matter that I know I'm crying for some totally different reason.
> CARMEL: Was it worse at any particular time?
> DELLA: Well I don't know. Yes probably before a period. I could just cry at anything. If I was tired I would get really impatient and I would have one day when I'd get really tired beforehand. I could accept that I would be emotionally fragile and it wasn't really stressful.

Six of the women commented on increasing forgetfulness but were uncertain whether to attribute it to menopause or ageing. However all agreed it was an embarrassment and a concern in terms of work and a competent image. Janet said:

> Yes I didn't feel I forgot anything [before] but sometimes now it will happen. Like we were told that . . . on Wednesday we [were] going to have a fellow come and talk to us on discipline. And then Wednesday afternoon I'm ready to go home . . . somebody [came by] and [said] 'Are you coming with me?' and I said 'Where are we going to?' 'Oh' I said, 'I forgot all about that.' I will remember as soon as they say it . . .

Helen relates a very similar incident but adds 'when you don't remember when reminded that's when it gets really scary'.

On further questioning all the women acknowledged that they had always had excellent memories and rarely needed to consult a diary. Karla made the comment that she had always noted men were not so concerned with forgetfulness at any age and 'probably left it up to women, wives or secretaries to do their remembering for them'. Neither, it is worth noting, do men have the physical marker of menopause to tie their possible increasing forgetfulness to. Twelve months on all commented that they were not having memory problems at work, but this might be due to learning to use a diary more efficiently.

Controlling the body

Most of these women implied that if the body is to work for you it must be controlled. Body control is something with which the pre-menopausal woman has had plenty of experience. There is a link, noted by Maureen, between controlling fertility and controlling the menopausal body by the use of HRT. Again it is worth noting this was unsolicited information. When thinking and talking about midlife the women talked of contraception. The pill, intra-uterine contraceptive devices (IUDs), abortions and sterilisations featured in a number of the women's stories. Three women appeared unhappy with contraceptive measures and referred to them in terms of being for 'the good of the family' or 'for the sake of the marriage or relationship'. In their descriptions of decisions taken with regard to controlling fertility, pragmatism is mixed with ambivalence, but overriding everything is the knowledge that fertility must be controlled. Other women in the study appeared happy with contraceptive choices.

The medical discourse touted the contraceptive pill as a means of controlling fertility and the feminists of the sixties and seventies hailed it as a form of liberation for women (Firestone 1970; Greer 1970). This is an example of two radically different groups sharing similar ideas, although from different perspectives, about contraception. It was only in the 1980s that feminists began to question the role of social agents in the marketing of the contraceptive pill and the minimal research carried out prior to its release (Bell 1986).

Beryl describes her decision to have an abortion with her fourth pregnancy as a pragmatic one which was best for all the family:

> It was a good idea really. It was best for everyone. I'd used the pill as contraception, except while I was in Malaysia. I had an IUD put in by a British doctor who didn't really know how to do it. It was very painful. That was removed and I had the third child in England. Then I had another loop put in, and when we were about to set off for a couple of months travelling on the way home I found I was pregnant with [our] third child only 14 months old, so I had an abortion because with the diseases and the loop and so on I wouldn't care to run the risk with the pregnancy or the baby. At the initial visits to the hospital, prior to the abortion of course, whoever I saw thought 'Oh yes not a good idea to have a loop in there and the pregnancy and the diseases and all that sort of thing.' But by the time it came around to the abortion they were saying 'What do you want an abortion for?' . . . It was about ten weeks by this time but I wasn't caught up in feeling pregnant and I treated it like a break in a contraceptive method. At the end I was very conscious though of their disapproval but I knew it was for the best.

Beryl also speaks of the pressure that was later put on her to have a tubal ligation following her fourth delivery by Caesarean section:

> Yes as a means of contraception because the gynaecologist wasn't happy with any more Caesareans, although it can be done. Particularly as with every one I went into labour . . . So I had a tubal ligation and again . . . I just didn't want to have that. I just felt that I didn't want to take the pill any longer either, but I just feel that it's one of those issues we really hear so much about where it's convenient for them [doctors].

Ingrid speaks of a tubal ligation at the age of 28 after the birth of her two sons as 'having more to do with the state of my marriage than anything else'. While quite happy with her decision at the time and for some years after, she regretted it following her divorce and during a five-year relationship. She said she wanted a child during the relationship or at least the ability to choose.

Karla, who had a sterilisation but at age 38, gives a similar reason for her decision:

> KARLA: I knew my marriage wouldn't have survived a third child. It didn't survive anyway (laughs).
> CARMEL: Did you want another child?
> KARLA: Yes. I think so.

Karla said she regretted having a sterilisation and felt 'like a spayed cat'. She reflects on this as a 'gut feeling' rather than rejection at an intellectual level and as something she had not anticipated. Karla's husband ended the marriage four years after the sterilisation and Karla considered it was at that time she mourned the third child she had never had. She returned to the issue of control over her body when recounting an embarrassing episode as a sessional lecturer:

> I vividly remember having a period and being quite oblivious and happy one minute as I was being introduced, got up to speak and flooded. I sat down again and gave the talk seated. I don't know what they thought. All I could think of was 'how am I going to get to the bathroom from here'. It doesn't do a lot for your confidence or image. You feel that you no longer have control over your body.

Emily Martin (1987), drawing on Goffman's (1971) classic study of presentation of self, has theorised in relation to menopausal symptoms, namely hot flushes, that women suffer primarily from embarrassment and it is the perception of others that affects them most. The embarrassment is compounded by their often lower status in work and social situations. I don't think this is the whole story. Women in this study were less concerned with others' opinions and more concerned with measuring up to their own mental picture of what constitutes a professional and competent image.

Maureen expresses resentment at 'doing all those thing to my body for the sake of a man'. She had taken the pill for a number of years while married and, subsequent to her divorce, during a five year relationship with a younger man. She had a sterilisation, aged 48, at his insistence. Although she acknowledges her fertility was coming to an end she believes the sterilisation made a difference to how she felt about her body:

> I never felt the same after it. Prior to the sterilisation my body felt richly fertile and very sexual and then I started, within three months, to have night sweats, my periods became irregular and light. No one warned me.

Perhaps women in a relationship can never have an autonomous attitude to their body. Foucault (1981) contends that the way in which discourse constitutes the mind and body is always part of a wider network of power relations, often with institutional bases. These include medicine, social welfare, education, religion, organisation of the family and work. Women's bodies became subject to modern science from the beginning of the eighteenth century. Not only did this have the effect of ascribing pathology to them, but it also placed the responsibility of ensuring fecundity with women. This has been modified with the advent of the contraceptive pill and other methods of contraception, which ensure a controlled fertility that fulfils the responsibility to the family without impinging on the need for the majority of women to work. At the same time there is still the expectation that they will be the primary carers of young children. The ageing baby boomers and an increasing incidence of divorce mean more emphasis on control in midlife. That is, more women are likely to be single parents with the primary financial responsibility for young children in midlife. One of the means of achieving control and managing the midlife body is by opting for HRT.

The continuing focus on controlling the female body via medical and scientific means extends into midlife with HRT playing a part in constructing menopause and, by extension, the midlife body. Barbara had very few menopausal symptoms and tells a funny story that typifies the way in which the biomedical model and HRT have become integral to perceptions of midlife and menopause, but also demonstrates that the general practitioner is not always the main exponent of this approach:

So I thought since I'm hearing all these things about menopause and hormones I'd better go to the doctor [a family doctor of many years standing]. I went in and said 'Should I be taking hormones?' And he said 'Have you got this and have you got that?' and I said 'No', and he said 'Get out of here.'

The experiences of Deidre and Jill are also interesting. Both women reported to their general practitioners symptoms they now consider were consistent with menopause. Jill experienced severe premenstrual tension, irregular periods and hot flushes. Menopausal symptoms commenced following the death of her mother. She was also experiencing marital difficulties:

> Well I mean at the time I couldn't get a doctor to admit I was menopausal. I felt I was. I felt that it was happening and even after mother died, as I said, the doctor thought it was more the grieving process.

Deidre reported irregular periods, flooding, a continual vaginal discharge and extreme tiredness:

> I can remember at Cook Town one night, I gave this lecture. Luckily I was standing up, had the white habit on I might tell you, and had this great flood. So when everybody was having supper I just ran home. Luckily the car seat covers, you could take off and wash. So you are away from home and you sort of feel 'Oh well. I don't know what this is but I presume it is just the effect of being away.'

Deidre, as a result of a continuing vaginal discharge had taken to wearing a tampon continuously. Both women had hormone levels taken and were told they were not menopausal according to the test results. Guillemin (1994) has argued that the use of tools such as blood tests acts to define a woman's experience as normal or abnormal, and then to further classify the origin of any abnormality, assessing whether it can be categorised as due to a hormone deficiency. In the case of Deidre and Jill this operated to deny their own experience. Like women using obstetric services studied by Anne Oakley (1980), they found only the doctors' observations were relevant.

Deidre reported a litany of symptoms experienced over a two-year period resulting in inappropriate treatment for monilia (thrush) trichomoniasis and finally a severe reaction to the last of a series of antibiotic treatments. In desperation she went to a women's clinic connected to a public hospital where she was not known:

> I then took myself off to [the clinic] in disguise and had the first proper physical examination, including a vaginal examination, by this lovely woman doctor who discovered I had a tampon in place that must have been there for ages. By this time [several years] the worst of menopause had been and gone.

The degree of choice exercised by women in commencing or ceasing HRT was variable, at least initially. However the majority of women in the study did not come across as mindless dupes. The influence of social discourse on bodily experience was evident in the women's reflection on choices they had made and the ongoing monitoring they were engaged in to ascertain the response of their bodies to HRT.

Jill said her reasons for taking HRT initially, once she was acknowledged as menopausal, related to relief of symptoms and the desire to regain some control:

> ... but now [2 years on] ... hormone replacement therapy is great. I actually made the decision and the hormone replacement therapy, the real turning point on it, was not the hormone replacement therapy for menopause [once symptoms were under control] but more for [protection against] osteoporosis and cardiovascular disease.

Like Jill, those women who chose to take HRT, or were contemplating it, saw it initially as a means of taking control, usually in order to manage their lives, particularly their working lives. It was only later that they paid attention to the issues surrounding HRT. No women reported taking it to delay ageing.

Karla, who at the second interview had commenced HRT, had, like Jill, explored the literature for and against it. She considers that it has helped in the short term, most particularly with overcoming tiredness and enabling her to cope with the myriad of demands on her. However she does not see it as a long-term choice and appears more influenced by feminist literature highlighting the potential dangers of long-term HRT use: 'I'm just a bit concerned about the latest studies linking long-term HRT use to an increased risk of breast cancer . . . ' For some such as Joanne it was just one of the range of options. She also meditates, exercises regularly, takes calcium and vitamin supplements, and does yoga.

Della typifies a woman in the process of making up her mind about HRT. Capturing some aspects of this process was made possible by following the women for twelve months. Della, just prior to the first interview, was referred by her general practitioner to a gynaecologist because of her irregular periods and was prescribed HRT. She revealed in the first interview a family history of breast and uterine cancer. When asked if the doctor prescribing HRT had taken a health history including factors such as these Della said no; she seemed puzzled and angry at the reasons the gynaecologist had given for prescribing HRT:

> DELLA: He said with your periods being every six weeks, you are not ovulating. He said something else. I said well what the hell do I want to ovulate for at my age and stage in life. And he sort of looked at me as if I was ridiculous. Whether I was or not was irrelevant but he was making some assumptions about me.
> CARMEL: From being four weekly [periods] or whatever?
> DELLA: Yes. And anyway there were some polyps and stuff and I mean it wasn't a big issue and I really kind of resented going onto hormone replacement therapy for some reason or other.
>
> I think it was a weight issue too. Because I had previously lost 20 kilos and . . . he then wanted to up the dose and I resisted and said I don't want you to and he didn't. Because I felt alright as I was. But I was definitely aware of my emotional instability in my cycle especially before menstruating . . .

Della demonstrates a resistance to HRT and anger at the lack of information and respect displayed by the gynaecologist. She expresses a need to know at what stage she is at in terms of menopause and what would be normal for her without HRT:

> CARMEL: So have you thought about going off it [HRT].
> DELLA: Yes. Accidentally I didn't take my provera this month and I had a period the day after I was supposed to have it. The really interesting thoughts that I had were, 'If I'm on HRT I don't know if I'm normal.'
> . . . Then I thought I'm still having them because I'm me and I'm

working in a normal [way], whatever normal is, and it is not just a chemically induced period.

Della then went on to add up the pros and cons of being on HRT for protection against osteoporosis and relief of symptoms versus what she perceived as her greater risk of dying of uterine cancer like her mother. By the time of the second interview she had decided to continue with the therapy for the time being. She still expresses doubts about HRT from the perspective of control, but acknowledges that she is experiencing symptoms that may or may not be helped by HRT:

> CARMEL: Is it a troubling time generally?
> DELLA: Yes and I keep asking 'Do I have control or the doctors?'

Another reason for taking HRT related to asserting control of a different kind. Maureen was in a relationship with a younger man at the time of the onset of menopause and said she did not want him to know she was menopausal: 'I started to have hot flushes at night and G. said "Is that tropical thing you had recurring?" and I said "Yes." I didn't want him to know I was menopausal and all that might mean.'

The relationship had ceased three months prior to the first interview. Reflecting back on a relationship with no real emotional security Maureen was conscious of being stereotyped as ageing and no longer desirable. She considered HRT beneficial in terms of libido and a means of giving her more control in a relationship with a younger man. She related carrying out a little experiment to check the efficacy of HRT:

> CARMEL: You said you thought you were going off sex [once menopausal]. Did HRT help?
> MAUREEN: Yes. I tried an experiment once to check this out. I took twice the recommended dose. I had such a heightened libido I could have raped the tramdriver.

Toni sees HRT as beneficial for the opposite reason to that given by Maureen at the first interview. A particularly distressing menopausal symptom Toni reported at the second interview was heightened libido. On being asked how she was relative to twelve months ago she said:

I'm much worse than I was 12 months ago . . . irritability, tiredness, hot flushes and now hormones all over the place. I'm horny all the time. It's just awful. I remember reading this book about a nymphomaniac who committed suicide and I can understand why.

Toni had been to her general practitioner and had an appointment to visit a menopause clinic. Because of Toni's acute distress I telephoned her several months after her visit to the clinic. She had commenced HRT and was happy to report an overall improvement in her general well-being, most particularly a normal libido.

Janet is the only women whose situation approximates that decried by feminist critics: one where she has handed over control and could be said to have been made totally dependent on her general practitioner and the pharmaceutical companies. At the age of 42 she visited her (male) general practitioner and complained of tiredness and a lack of interest at work. She was diagnosed as depressed and prescribed anti-depressants. Six years later she is still taking them and on attempting to wean herself off them was castigated by her doctor and told she had a chemical deficit and must take them for life. Similarly, with the onset of mild menopausal symptoms at the age of 48, between the first and second interview, she was prescribed HRT and told she must take it for life.

LISTENING TO THE BODY

Anne, Margaret and Georgie after being prescribed HRT had taken it for periods varying from six months to four years and had then chosen to cease it. With the exception of Margaret they saw it as beneficial in the short term and as a way of helping them cope with responsibilities. Margaret chose to cease it because of adverse reactions and in order 'to own my menopause'. Her general practitioner was quite happy to support her in this decision.

Anne and Georgie made a decision to cease HRT and used very similar terms when recording this decision in their diaries. Anne wrote 'I began to think, no, it's not right for me. Why am I putting it in my body?' She had become aware of symptoms 'like the worst

PMT' when on the progesterone cycle and was later (two months after ceasing HRT) diagnosed with endometriosis. Anne also noted in her diary, and at the second interview, being influenced by reading *Menopause without Medicine* by Linda Ojeda. Georgie recorded in her diary: 'I think my body is trying to tell me something. I've decided not to take HRT this cycle to see if the progesterone is compounding the depression or vice versa.' Two months later she wrote, 'The night sweats are back but I'm happy with my decision not to continue with HRT. I'm not comfortable putting that in my body.'

Responding to the body is also reflected in Margaret's decision to cease HRT:

> I went off it because I felt awful, as though I didn't own my body. I felt bloated, my breasts felt tender . . . I was Sally schizophrenic. I was quite crazy. Since I went off it I don't feel that way. I just generally feel awful (laughs).

Both Anne and Georgie visited a Chinese herbalist after ceasing HRT (coincidentally the same one). They professed to be happier trying a therapy which aimed at 'bringing the body into balance rather than prescribing something long term'.

At the time of the second interview Maureen discussed both her reasons for staying on HRT and her desire to cease it. Her reasons for staying on HRT related to her state of health and the stress of dealing with her mentally ill son. Her desire to cease it related to a desire to be in touch with her body and to experience it in an age-appropriate way:

> CARMEL: And you would personally prefer not to be on HRT. You see no reason to be on it?
> MAUREEN: No, I don't. Except that I'm a bit afraid to go off it. I want to see what sort of person I'd be without it. It's like I'm being kept as a perpetual teenager, that's how I see it. As if you gave teenagers some hormone in order that they didn't reach puberty.
> CARMEL: So you see menopause as a physical developmental stage as well as an emotional and psychological one.
> MAUREEN: Yes it is, well it should be . . . Oh and the other thing about it is I don't know but it appears to be stimulating in terms of making you feel randy.

CARMEL: Everything you're saying suggests that there may be a time for everything and continuing to take HRT makes you feel 'out of sync'.
MAUREEN: To be feeling randy at my age, and without a partner, is not an enjoyable thing. You know the classic old things: that randy old bitch and the idea that's been around of the old women out of control.

Jane, by the time of the second interview, had been taking HRT for fourteen months and saw it as beneficial but as something she would monitor, 'I'm happy to take it for the time being.' Helen, after eighteen months of therapy was 'very happy with HRT' and considered it had played a role in assisting her to cope with the demands of her job. Karla was considering ceasing HRT. She had also noted periods of depression that coincided with taking progesterone.

It is apparent that Jill's, Karla's, Georgie's, Margaret's and Anne's decisions were influenced by information gleaned from texts on menopause and general reading in the area of menopause. For example Margaret's desire to 'own her own menopause' reflects Germaine Greer's thesis in *The Change*, a book she acknowledges as influential. Anne's decision was aided by reading of alternative approaches to managing menopause. Jill reached her decision after weighing up all the evidence, primarily gleaned from medical journals, along with feeling comfortable about taking HRT.

VIEWING THE BODY

Viewing the body refers to the relationship women had with their bodies and how they perceived their bodies over time. While not all women who had never married ignored their bodies and pushed themselves in a physical sense, a less than accepting and comfortable relationship with their bodies was demonstrated. Anne said that 'I used to say "Well why should I have a uterus when it's not going to be used?", especially when I was having a bad menstrual cycle.'

Della resented both the pain and inconvenience of menstruation, particularly as a celibate woman:

I used to bitterly resent bleeding every month. That really pissed me off. It was so inconvenient and after all for no purpose. I hated it. Initially I used to get all these cramps and pain and stuff and I thought it was normal. I couldn't stand up sometimes in school. I went to a chiropractor and he put my hip back which was out and I had periods without pain for the first time at 34. But I still hated and resented them and part of that was the hygiene that was practised when I was at boarding school where we had cloth napkins that we had to wash out and it was revolting . . . finally getting to use tampons was a turning point as was seeing [a psychologist].

In keeping with the experience of some women and their lack of basic understanding of their bodies, the swinging sixties notwithstanding, is Toni's story. She reports a childhood and adolescence with an abusive father and a loving but undemonstrative mother who provided no sex education. She attended a Catholic same-sex school:

Well, you see Mum is very straight-laced and non-touching and non-verbal. Mum just can't cope with having to pat your head or anything like that. When it came time to tell everybody about the birds and the bees, Mum said, I can't do it, and they all fell pregnant and had to get married.

Toni later recounted her experience of dating in her late teens and later becoming pregnant (although taking the pill) to a married man. On discovering she was pregnant she took herbal remedies, obtained by her friend, in order to procure an abortion. She aborted alone and at night. Several years later, following ongoing problems, she had a dilatation and curettage. She did not inform her lover of the pregnancy or the abortion.

Helen's experience, while different from Toni's in many respects, also reflects a lack of understanding and valuing of the sexual body, and a lack of comfortable relationships with the opposite sex in adolescence, to say nothing of the constraints placed on young women in the early 1960s. She also attended a same-sex school (Anglican). Her relationship with her father was and is problematic. He is a domineering man who 'look[s] down on females'. Her first sexual relationship in her late twenties was with a separated/divorced man who told her 'We have to accept we're second best.'

It was only a number of years later she realised that 'He was telling me more about himself, projecting his own inadequacies on to me.'

Ingrid expressed some regret at the ambivalence she experienced when pregnant and as a young mother and attributes this, as a feminist, to fighting against 'the whole biological determinism thing'. In so doing she considers she missed out on some of the potential benefits pregnancy and small childen can bring to women:

> I don't know but I wonder for me if it hasn't got something to do with the experiences of my — our—generation. In the late sixties early seventies if you had the experiences I had, you had to put your sexuality and your reproductivity aside. I had my children quite young. I never mentioned them in public. I kept my private and my public life quite separate. People knew me for months before they knew I had children. They were shocked when they came to my place for dinner and found two young kids. It wasn't fashionable in the circles I moved [in]. I can remember going to women's groups with F in the basket and I was the only woman there with a child. I mean I was heterosexual, I was married (not living with someone), I had two children and I lived in the suburbs. I mean how straight. It was during the period of that whole reaction to women's biological determinism. At one level I enjoyed it but at another level you had to keep it quiet. I think women today are able to go full bore with the reproductive thing. I met a young woman recently. There was something lush about her. I mean she was intelligent, she was academic.

Karla, also a woman who considered herself heavily influenced by feminism in the late 1960s and early 1970s, expresses a similar sense of enjoying balancing everything but at the same time looks back with some regret. She notes that it was a point of pride for her that she worked almost until her children were born and 'had one day off sick for the two pregnancies'. She does, however, state wistfully:

> I was so busy proving I could do it all I had little time to really enjoy it . . . We were the generation who bought the message that not only could you have it all but you were expected to do it all. At best my ex-husband only paid lip service to the equality thing and certainly did very well out of it. I suppose if I had achieved the successful marriage in midlife I would say it was worth it. At the moment I just feel

physically exhausted. I do think it is possible to wear out! I mean I compare myself with my mother at this age (46). She was doing better on every level — she certainly thinks she was. Mind you I'm not saying for a minute that I wanted to be dependent on a man.

At the same time the women who were divorced but had experienced years of a partnership or partnerships appeared more at home with their bodies while still expressing some ambivalence. For several women this was expressed in terms of their understanding of their bodies, in a sexual way. Ingrid expresses this relationship with her body and the opposite sex in terms of her ability to attract men and the power this gave her:

INGRID: I've always been very attractive. In social situations there's always been that sort of play, that chemistry. I'm not big-noting myself. You just go into a social situation and there's always that anonymous play and you just catch someone's eye. I've always been that sort of person.
CARMEL: So you've always related strongly to men.
INGRID: But not in an easy way. There's always been that antagonism and the men I've been attracted to have always been intellectual, quirky, artistic . . . Putting aside involvement though, I've always had, as part of my life, in the public space, a kind of play, a physical play with men . . . I've always got off on desire.
CARMEL: In terms of a sense of antagonism in relationships — did you want to retain your autonomy?
INGRID: Yes, but I don't think it was entirely a power thing. It's not as clear as that. I think it might have something to do with the man–woman thing. There has always been an edge in all my relationships or even in those attractions in the public space. A power which attracted me. I didn't understand it when I was younger. I think there is an enormous amount of power and a high degree of control for women in this.

The downside of being in touch with the body in a sexual sense is the realisation that a relationship depends on a potential partner responding and this may not be a given in midlife. Ingrid expresses this in terms of coming to accept a loss:

Sexuality has been a very strong part of my life. I've taken it for granted. At times now I'm quite haunted by its loss, devastated by it. It's a very powerful thing and I've always taken it for granted . . . you don't think about it intellectually. It's been a given. It's only now I realise the power of it because it's on the way out.

Lynne Segal (1992), in a revealing and very personal essay on sexuality, explores female desire and pleads for theoretical explorations by feminists of the links between sex and power and sex and gender that go beyond naive explanations (namely that men are by nature sexually aggressive and coercive and that women need only rediscover their own natural sexuality). While acknowledging that sexual behaviours are culturally and historically specific what is needed is a clearer understanding of what feeds our desires, that is, 'how sexual desire comes to express such a variety of other social needs: needs which are irrational, unconscious and not easily understood' (p. 127). Segal makes the point that to assume that all male sexuality is about power and dominance, and all female sexuality is bland, is shortsighted and wrong. What is interesting in Ingrid's account of her previous relationships is the sense of regret that there was this feeling of antagonism that resulted in 'a meanness in my relationships'. It suggests reflection on the degree to which she may have internalised the feminist message that in order to retain her autonomy she must hold something back. However well this may have worked for her at the time she now feels a sense of regret. This demonstrates the complexity in sexual relationships and the way in which perceptions of the body are influenced by sexuality and sexual experience.

Rebecca also expresses her relationship to her body in a sexual sense and the part played by an awareness of her body as attractive in sexual relationships. Rebecca is without a full-time partner and is expressing disgust with an ageing body and flirting with the idea of a face-lift:

> CARMEL: You spoke quite graphically about catching sight of your body in the window on getting out of the pool and that's something you prefer...
> REBECCA: Well there's this tummy now, there's this cut [recent operation scar] and there's this, that you know I've always prided myself on a good figure...

CARMEL: And all of a sudden it's beyond your control?
REBECCA: Yes . . . and even with all this exercise . . . it's all soft, you know. Yes, I'd love to have a facelift, love to.
CARMEL: Why?
REBECCA: Well I'd like to look in the mirror and like what I see but also I don't want to spend the rest of my life alone.

The difference between Ingrid and Rebecca appears to be in the way Rebecca objectifies her body. Whereas Ingrid expresses the power her sexuality afforded her there is no sense of her body as 'the object of the gaze' — she is very much in control of the interaction. While she expresses a sense of loss of a youthful and sexually attractive body there is also the acceptance of the inevitability of time. The lack of a current male partner does not appear to be a major concern for her. In fact Ingrid makes it clear that in midlife she prefers the company of women and that her female friends meet most of her social needs. At the same time she remains interested in the possibility of further relationships: 'It's two years since I had a screw and I'd hate to think that was the last time (laughs) . . . '

Rebecca on the other hand sees the lack of a partner as the major problem in her life. She contends she would get over the breakup of her second marriage quite rapidly if another compatible partner came along. Twelve months later she professes that she is much happier since her recent (three-months standing) involvement in a relationship. Wendy Hollway (1984) has theorised that the degree of 'investment' in a particular position often reflects how much an individual perceives they can get out of it. Rebecca undoubtedly sees a partner as essential to any sort of life.

Joanne, a divorced woman, appears very much in tune with her body. She relates this to having been a gymnast and a dancer. Her relationship with her body and the way in which she views her body influences the way she approaches ageing and menopause. The era in which Joanne came of age did not emphasise the importance of exercise and fitness, and the norm for the majority of women was to abandon any regular participation in sport and exercise once children came along:

CARMEL: So how do you feel about ageing in a physical sense? Is that something that . . .

JOANNE: Well, because of my background being a physical education teacher and a dancer, I am very aware of my body and also I have an attitude to it that I can make changes in my body. I am in control of my body, and I suppose well I've had one menopausal experience and I could sense that I could have easily slipped into what happened to my body after I'd had a child, which is my body's getting away from me. Saying, alright let's give in to it, age has taken over or I've become a real women now . . . but I don't let that happen. And so each time I had a child I would say 'right I can get back the figure and the energy that I had before' and you know, I make an effort, and once I have got back to my normal weight and my normal amount of physical ability you know, I just steady up and I'd be there again, my metabolism is back to what it was before. So this time when I had all the hot flushes and things I paid particular attention to diet and exercise . . .

While Joanne speaks of being in control of her body it is in the sense of being in tune with her body rather than ignoring the body or making it work for her in potentially injurious ways. At the same time her choice of words 'I've become a real woman now' is interesting and conjures up a Victorian notion of womanhood. Two competing discourses appear to be at work, the soft, womanly body versus the fit and toned body. Susan Bordo (1992), citing Kim Chernin, has identified 'the tyranny of slenderness' and the androgynous, adolescent, athletic body type as a post-sixties phenomenon. Bordo identifies Marilyn Monroe as the dominant ideal body type of the 1950s and comments on the change in perception of the ideal body type by noting that one of her students in the early 1990s referred to Marilyn Monroe as 'a cow'. Joanne as an athlete/dancer appears to have identified with the athletic body but acknowledges the still competing discourse of the soft, womanly body of the mother. Embodiment for Joanne was further influenced by her experience as a dancer and gymnast. Pierre Bordieu's (1992) notion of bodily praxis as a mode of knowledge is useful for understanding Joanne's identification at the level of the body. Working in an anthropological context Bordieu has theorised that the body engages with the environment or the material world and acquires a form of knowledge that is below the level of consciousness and is to an extent opposed to conscious memory and knowledge. He contends that 'the body is constantly mingled with all the knowledge it produces' (p. 73). For Joanne her knowledge at the bodily level was a factor in deciding against giving in to becoming 'a real woman' — a continuing influence in how she approaches midlife and menopause.

Ingrid, while comfortable with her body in a sexual sense, acknowledges her tendency to ignore the body and 'not take care of it'. She smokes and as a women alone, along with Barbara and Margaret, speaks of involvement in hard physical activity as necessary, as leisure and as pleasurable. Ingrid, for example, speaks with pride of laying all the bricks in her garden. Barbara and Margaret also take great pride in doing all the manual labour around their houses including laying bricks, carting sacks and fixing tiles on the roof. Margaret comments that the ageing body doesn't allow her to do what she once did, but in not looking after her body (she also smokes) she has contributed to its decline. All three women blame themselves for any structural damage they may have done to their bodies. The notion of self-care and responsibility is evident here even if these women, as women alone, may have had little choice in 'working the body' this way.

In a few cases the fight to achieve a slim body is referred to, also reflecting the post-1960s discourse. Margaret considers that her life has been a round of diets, an approach that no longer works in midlife. Winnie, prior to midlife, was never happy with her body shape and dieted in an attempt to achieve a slim body. As a 48-year-old midlife woman currently in a relationship with a man twenty years younger she is very happy with her body:

> Oh yes [in the past] I thought I was huge and had too much in the wrong places. Thighs and legs too big and not enough bust. But now I like my body. I've met a couple of younger men too, which was a surprise because I wasn't looking for that. They see me as a sexually desirable person.

Achieving a more comfortable relationship with one's body in midlife appears to be a process to be worked through, which in some cases is facilitated by a body that is no longer perceived as unpredictable. For example, Alice had a hysterectomy and both ovaries removed in her early forties. Her experiences of painful periods and undiagnosed endometriosis enabled her, following a transient sense of loss, to see the procedure as very positive for her health and the way she related to her body: 'I mean suddenly I could feel at ease with my body because it wasn't doing all those unpredictable things any more.' Sigrid too, diagnosed with uterine cancer, welcomed a hysterectomy as both necessary and lifesaving but also as a means of ending painful periods.

There is also the sense of loss of the youthful self to work through and this is expressed by Ingrid:

> Well I realised I was no longer in my twenties . . . I think there has been a dramatic difference in my appearance since 40. The ageing process seems to have accelerated. I look in the mirror and try out all these different poses and I'll play with images. You know what I mean. There's a whole lot of stuff I've done to try and reconcile . . . sometimes I'm quite devastated by the loss.

Karla remembers looking down one day 'and seeing my mother's feet'. She recalls this as significant in acknowledging her ageing and 'in a funny sort of way a sense of continuity'.

While aware of the emphasis on body and beauty maintenance few women appear unduly influenced by it. Irritable comments about 'inappropriate role models' and 'the body police' and 'that pumped-up lycra set' indicate resistance to the beauty myth. This contrasts with Rebecca's desire to have a face-lift in order to feel better about herself and be able to attract a man.

Coming to terms with ageing is a continual process that resembles the grieving process. The diaries demonstrate good days and bad days. There are several references to the body as an old car 'just needing to get into gear'. There are also references to 'lumps and bumps popping up everywhere' and 'veins popping out' as well as comparing notes of physical decline with other women at social functions. The notion of an ongoing process is captured by Anne. Having thought she had come to terms with being middle-aged she suddenly found herself, at 54, being treated as an old lady:

It must be the grey hair but people started giving me seats in buses when I was away [on holidays] and if I asked the way taking my arm and calling me dear. When I came back I went into Myer's and because they'd rearranged the shop I got thoroughly disoriented and thought 'they're right I'm a bumbling old lady' . . . I can laugh about it now.

Ageing is not a process that is greeted with relish. It is, however, greeted with humour and variations on the theme 'ask me again in a year'. I'll leave the last word to Barbara: 'I don't care how miserable everybody else wants to be. I intend to live to be a hundred, have a good time and be a nuisance to everyone. I'm not just getting older I'm getting better!'

DISCOURSE INFLUENCING EXPERIENCE

THE MIND–BODY DIVIDE AND FEMINIST DISCOURSE

The separation of mind and body and the domination of the body by the mind influenced middle-aged women coming of age. As Susan Bordo (1992) has identified, the separation of mind and body is a consistent theme in Western thought from Plato to Augustine. An image that occurs in Plato, Descartes and Augustine is that of the body as a prison or as a form of confinement. Plato depicted the body as alien, as not self; Descartes represented the body as a machine needing to be dominated by the mind; and Augustine saw the body as the enemy and stressed the need to control the flesh or the body. Added to this was the challenge by feminists in the late 1960s and the early 1970s to biological determinism. If women were to be seen as equal to men the biology as destiny argument needed to be challenged and in fact what was posited was 'androgyny', a social situation transcending gender. For women in the 1970s a combination of the puritan denial of the body and a feminist discourse that sought to deconstruct the notion of the female sex as the inferior sex set up the ideal conditions for denial of the body. At the very least bodily functions were seen as subservient to the mind. Emily Martin (1987) theorised in relation to women, menopause, menstruation and childbirth that the body in medical texts (and therefore as part of medical discourse) was organised as a hierarchical system and inherent in this concept was the mind controlling the body.

Women in the study, particularly single women exemplified by Alice and Georgie, internalised these messages (as no doubt did men), in terms of making the body 'work for you'. At the same time they attempted to ignore the reality of menstruation. Another discourse, that of the feminists, while setting out to challenge the negative aspects of biological determinism also set up the situation for a denial of the feminine body in terms of its functions (menstruation, pregnancy, motherhood and heterosexual sexuality) within a patriarchal context. Ingrid, in describing the way she kept her life as a wife and mother in the private sphere compartmentalised from her feminist activities, is an example of what Sandra Coney (1993, p. 35) describes as 'a woman caught on the cusp of the old world and the new'. The influence of feminist discourse also spilled over into Ingrid's relationships with men. She considers that in attempting to retain her autonomy there was a 'meanness in her relationships'. This reflects the problem of the heterosexual female caught up in a feminist culture. Karla, who as a young woman was also heavily influenced by feminist discourse, has a sense of 'being gypped' by a prevailing message (to have and do it all), which has nonetheless left her at midlife perceiving herself as poorer in an emotional, physical and financial sense than her own mother. Maureen in retrospect sees her relationships with men as dominated by the need to control her fertility and resents 'doing all those things to my body for the sake of a man'. At the same time she is mourning the loss of a lover and a sense of family and maintains she would do it all again to achieve or maintain a successful relationship.

Beryl expresses resentment with a male-dominated medical profession that attempted to make decisions for her in relation to her body, reflecting the influence of medical discourse. This influence is also apparent in the reasons some of the women give for continuing to take HRT. At the same time alternative points of view also influence long-term decision-making regarding HRT. The most consistent reason for taking HRT, particularly in the short term, is for control. Once control is achieved, alternative approaches to managing menopause tend to be investigated.

Rosalind Coward (1983, 1984) and others have explored the impact of the dominant discourse of the patriarchal family on women as they attempt to negotiate life, work and sexuality. Women still desire a fulfilling relationship. Not all ever achieve this and some, such as the divorced women in my study, perceive themselves as having lost it and, in reflection like Karla, consider the odds may have been stacked against them anyway.

Rosalind Coward (1984), in exploring images of women, notes how pervasive the art of body maintenance became in the 1970s and early 1980s after having been taken up by women's magazines. She sees it as little different from ideologies exhorting physical attractiveness and believes it is another way of disempowering women. Anthony Giddens (1991) has a more optimistic view and sees it as a way of taking control 'or cohering the self as an integrated whole'. Joanne touches on this with her references to two different discourses influencing her as a young mother and as a middle-aged woman. The old notion that motherhood brought a different set of expectations ('You are a woman now') and the new discourse that being a mother is no excuse to let yourself go ('trim, taut and terrific') applied to all age groups. Resistance to this latter view, often influenced by feminist writings, was expressed by the majority of women in the study.

The discourses in circulation are competing, for example, the medical versus the alternative view. Coward's (1984) notion of female desire and Hollway's (1984) notion of investment are similar. Coward sees female desire as constructed within a society that sustains male privilege. At the same time, we all desire rewarding relationships, the majority of women want children and will make the necessary compromises within a patriarchal culture. Hollway, in a similar vein, contends that investment in a particular position relates to how much an individual perceives they can get out of it. Women, such as Rebecca, will invest in what pays off. Some of course are luckier than others.

In concluding, this chapter has dealt with striving for wholeness or what Giddens has termed the reflexive project of self. I contend that the body is at the centre of this for women throughout their lives; whether it is attempting to ignore it as a celibate woman, controlling fertility as a partnered women, or controlling it and making it work as a midlife and menopausal woman. The strongest message to emerge from the women in this study was a sense of striving in midlife for wholeness and integration: *the* body becoming *my* body.

5
MAKING THE CHANGE

Lyn Richards

'The Change', as opposed to any other change, means one thing to Australian women. Menopause. The literature agrees on this and, as shown in chapter 3, there is a lot of literature. For this generation of women there is a clear message: of all the changes in women's changing lives, this one is nominated as 'the Change', and most inevitably as a negative transition.

Another message backs this one. For most women, the literature asserts, the Change will be experienced as one of many changes. Body changes will be related to, or trigger, other changes. While women's bodies are changing so too are their family and work lives, their partnerships, their social networks, their goals and ideas of themselves, and their perceptions of how they are seen in society. The cumulative picture is of chaos, everything changing at once, and always negatively — the ultimate, multiple transition. But this is a strange sort of change, marked by ambiguity and continuity, and it itself is changing.

It took us a long time to realise how unsatisfactory the metaphor of transition is for the experience of most midlife women. Trendy in social science, it is in the titles of many works on menopause and the text of more. 'Transition' is a word that implies, in the words of the *Oxford English Dictionary*, 'change, from one place or state or act or set of circumstances to another'.

The term carries two implications. A transition is a recognisable event. And once you have made a transition, you normally can't go back. To describe menopause as transition then is to imply it is an evident event and one which irrevocably changes a woman's life.

Looking back, I think we brought to the study the expectation that in our data menopause and midlife would be transition. And we found it there. This was for three very different reasons.

We found transition firstly because the literature on menopause persistently talks of transition. The assumption that menopause is a transition, even the *major* transition, in women's lives, is built into its nickname, celebrated in the title of the text most read by women we talked to (Greer 1991); and into medical and social research and popular literature (e.g. Dickson & Henriques 1988; Saltman 1994; Sheehy 1993). Secondly, we found transition in our data because our attention was held by the stories of a very few women who had taken control of their lives at menopause, using it as a time — or rather a time out — when they could rethink and redirect many aspects of their personal and social lives. They were unusual, and often unusually articulate, women for whom a number of midlife processes coincided, and who often were engaging with the discourse of transition in the critical literature.

We found transition thirdly because of who and where we were and what we heard. For each member of this team when the project began, menopause was yet to come, though some, including me, were nearing the age group. Unlike most women pre-menopause, who, our data showed, rarely think much about it, we were collecting and comparing a range of experiences. They provided a formidable line-up of physical or psychological problems. (The QSR NUD•IST computer program supports creation of new categories out of the data, and we collected categories for each of the physical or psychological 'symptoms' of menopause people related to us. The index system grew 30 nodes for different physical 'symptoms', 22 for psychological ones and 9 for other medical issues people associated with menopause — and not one of these was pleasant!) No woman of course experienced all sixty-one conditions, but from the many different experiences of the women we talked to, and the collected words of health advisers, we were building a negative cumulative picture of the coming 'event' that fitted no individual's experience. Perhaps more importantly, it was a picture that reflected the feelings of those women who feared that all these changes were permanent, that their bodies had altered irrevocably. By the end of the project we had balanced our expectations and the accounts of the literature with detailed accounts of women's agency and experiences in going *through* menopause, concluding that for most, however unpleasant the symptoms, it had been a break in the normal performance of their lives rather than a transition from one state to another.

Slowly, we came to the conclusion that menopause was a clear transition for very few women, and mostly they were the ones who chose to make it so. All women experienced some sense of change, temporary or permanent, at this time; but their experiences were widely varied, and very few were of a transition event that remade their lives.

What women did seem to experience in common was an interruption, sometimes critically serious, sometimes minimal, in their lives. Like the intermission in a play, it presented a break in continuity. How this was to be used was unclear, and the ways women used it varied according to their situations. However all intermissions end, you return to the theatre, and the play goes on.

This chapter focuses on change or non-change, and how this was anticipated, experienced and recalled. We learned from our data what we were learning from personal experience; that women differ greatly in the extent to which their lives change at midlife, and in the relevance of menopause to this change. We learned too that they vary in the extent to which they themselves feel they are directing, controlling or making those changes rather than merely being made by them.

Undoubtedly in our data some women saw no transition, some experienced the end of one part of their lives (with pleasure or despair), some determinedly avoided transition, and some took this opportunity to *make* the change. Any one woman might have several, even all, of these experiences. The following four sections scan that variety. In the first section, I explore the two areas of our data strongly indicating that menopause is not seen as a major transition — the survey responses from women of all ages and the accounts of mothers' experiences. The second section is about the different ways in which women felt something had ended: the end of menstruation, becoming old, the sense of losing control over the body, the empty nest. In the third section, the theme of the avoidance of transition by HRT is addressed. The fourth is about ways women worked at making midlife and menopause a transition, remaking their lives. It tells the story of one of the few women who found in midlife and menopause an opportunity to rethink, reassess, redirect, and take control.

WHAT CHANGE? WHEN THERE IS NO TRANSITION

We had two bodies of data that rebuked the assumption that menopause means transition. One was the survey; in that context, women talked about all sorts of changes — menopause featured for few as significant, and rarely as dominant. The other was data from women's memories of their mothers' experience. Mothers were almost uniformly pictured as having come through menopause, never as having been altered by it.

ONE LOT OF CHANGES AMONG MANY — WHAT THE SURVEY SAID

Our survey of women of all ages offered a chance to see the bigger picture. Our focus was on midlife. Simply to ask women for interviews about menopause is arguably to elevate it to an event. To avoid this we titled the survey 'Women's ideas of midlife'. No questions had been asked about menopause when respondents met a series of questions about change:
- What major changes do you see yourself currently going through?
- Which of these changes are positive for you?

- Are you concerned at any changes that you are currently experiencing?
- If so, which changes concern you?
- Do you see any changes that you are currently experiencing as bringing risks for you?
- If so, which changes are risky, and what are the risks?

The results were startling. A surprising number (nearly a third) did not offer any changes at all. A woman in her early fifties said, 'No changes, just progression.' Even more surprisingly, nearly two-thirds of the women in the 45–55 age bracket did not nominate menopause or associated changes or, if they did, did not nominate them as concerning. Only three seemed dominated by the changes of menopause. One of these, a woman in her early fifties, nominated as her major change, 'Moving into a new easier phase of life (apart from fatigue and menopause symptoms).' Her concerns? 'Extreme fatigue. Irritability and memory problems. Gaining weight.' Risks? 'Loss of family patience with forgetfulness and irritability.'

Those who did nominate change more often chose family changes. One wrote: '1. Moving to a smaller house. 2. Children leaving home. 3. Adjusting to a husband at home more.' The first and third of these she saw as positive. Another woman saw no positive changes:

> My feelings of emptiness e.g. no longer having a household. I get lonely even though I have a good husband. Since menopause I have felt angry, stressed, bored (not through inactivity, I lead a busy life). I just feel robbed of something I had before.

But determination showed when she was asked how she would handle the risks: 'Head on! One day at a time. I feel selfish and stupid. I must adjust and move with the times.'

Not only did few name major changes, very few offered pictures of transition — change from one thing to something else. Of these, the most vivid were not from midlife women: 'Giving up my full-time job and becoming a mother. It has been a big change for me. I have found it hard giving up my independence.'

Only 28% of the whole sample were concerned at changes they were experiencing. Women in their midlife years were slightly more likely to express concern about changes, but they were also more likely to nominate a lot of major changes, some positive. A woman in the 46–50 age bracket nominated four major changes: 'Children leaving. Approaching menopause. Husband considering retirement. Becoming Grandmother.' Of these, only the last was listed as a positive change. Another in the same age group mentioned 'early menopause' as a major change, but after 'giving up smoking'. Smoking was the positive change. Her concerns were, 'General tiredness. Slightly irritable.' Neither of these women saw risks.

Women in their late forties typically nominated many changes. If menopause appeared it was never positive, but it was rarely a cause of concern. Of the 86 women in this age group, only 12 mentioned menopause or another term for it in answer to the major changes question or the concern or risk questions. Of these, only three mentioned menopause and nothing else. More typical were answers like these to the major changes question:

> Menopause. Children all leaving home and only the youngest still with me.
>
> Greying hair and few wrinkles.
>
> Personal changes and societal i.e. major recession and increasing poverty and hardship for many people, also some ageing processes e.g. skin, hair, some weight gain.

A lot is happening to some of these women. Even for those currently experiencing menopause it does not get headline status. A professional woman in her late forties who worked full-time started menopause at 43 and experienced it as 'another challenge to overcome'. She chose the following words from the list of those given to describe menopause: tired, wisdom, stigma, relief, taking stock, freedom, journey. She was on HRT, felt she knew everything she needed to know about it, and expected to stay on it long-term. It 'stopped the hot flushes, improved my sleeping and aches and pains, increased energy, improved sex life'. Menopause here seems central. Yet earlier in the questionnaire when she was asked about major changes in her life she did not mention it: 'Major changes in work — becoming financially more difficult to make my practice a success. Have more significant role in work.' Her risks? 'I am more uncertain.' How would she handle risks? 'I will manage as always.'

A woman in a very different situation — divorced, low income, pre-menopausal — said, 'I don't foresee any problems.' She circled the word 'non-event' writing, 'People are much better informed, much less of a taboo subject'. Major changes for her were 'lifestyle, marital status, hopefully change of job'. Did she see any changes as bringing risks? 'Any change holds risks!' How would she handle them? She used the same phrase as the woman who felt 'robbed' — 'Head on if possible.'

'YOU GET THROUGH IT' — LEARNING FROM MOTHER

That menopause was no major change was a strong message in many of the open interviews. Those who saw it as no real change cited memories of their mothers' experience, or the confusion of their own, to interpret it as an intermission that passed, something you came through.

Mothers contributed to positive attitudes to menopause in two ways. Firstly, when comparing their lives with their mothers', almost all women agreed that menopause now held far less terror. And secondly, mothers were overwhelmingly remembered as 'coming through' it unchanged:

> I'd say perhaps people are becoming more informed and people are asking more questions and they are prepared to talk. Like a few years ago . . . I couldn't sit down and talk to you like this. And I don't think a lot of people would have because of social attitudes. Whereas now people are a lot more open. Therefore once things have come out in the open you don't suffer from the taboos and the mysterious mythology and whatever goes with these things.

Women agreed they were better informed than their mothers. We asked one group, 'Do you think the attitudes have changed since perhaps your mothers' day?' One woman said, 'I think in the era of my mother, "Oh, she's going through the Change", would be the constant comment. And, they'd forgive them anything because they were going through the Change.' Another laughed, 'Our mothers wouldn't have got in a group and talked about it would they? "Excuse me ladies. Tea or coffee?"' A third observed, 'I think women are hearing that it's alright to have changes, and seek advice, and treat themselves as best they can, and get on with life. I think it's a lot better than what my mother went through, where you were supposed to grin and bear it. "You'll get over it."' Everyone agreed that the subject was 'more open'.

Mothers feature strongly in our data, far more strongly, it seemed, than husbands. A search of the qualitative data for 'mother' or 'mum' retrieved over 7000 occurrences. (That comparative numbers can't be given for husbands and partners indicates the limitations of text search: unlike mothers they are usually named.) It was common for women to say they had never learned from their mothers, because 'then' such things could not be discussed. Yet all had learned something, gleaned from observations or impressions. What they learned often minimalised the drama. 'You get through it' was often the reported brief advice. It suggests continuity, not transition. You get through an obstacle course, or a tunnel, or passage, and then continue. Life goes on. About half of those who knew a bit about their mothers' experience had either gathered or were told by her that the experience was not a major or lasting one, and all the others assumed this: 'I had one of those mums that didn't tell you anything. They sort of went through it and I think that is where I got my ideas about it from.' Even when the mother was known to have had problems, the daughter had rarely set out to avoid the same experience. One woman had been rebuked by her mother for considering HRT:

> Her feeling is that it is interfering with nature and that menopause is a natural thing and all women must go through it despite the fact that it nearly drove her mad. I can remember it. She says that menopause is natural.

All women who mentioned their mothers' menopause seemed sure they had or would have much the same experience. The most common reason for this confidence was that they counted on having inherited characteristics guaranteeing they too would get through menopause easily:

> They say that, you know, daughters more or less take after their mothers. I knew that my mother hadn't started till her early fifties, so it never occurred to me that I might start earlier . . . Well, I don't think my mother had a lot of trouble with it . . . The thing most women seem to worry about are the terrible hot flushes . . . Well it didn't happen with Mum, so it probably won't happen with me either.

A second reason for confidence was simply that some knew little about their mothers' experience of menopause. Mothers had not discussed their experiences then, and now minimalised them:

> I think she must have been depressed because she was crying. Occasionally she would have this outburst saying 'Nobody loves me.' Then she would come and apologise and say . . . 'Look it is the change of life, OK?' . . . Then when I suggested to her that I think I am on the verge of becoming menopausal she said, 'Oh, you will be fine. You will have no trouble. None of us ever had any trouble' . . . I didn't say, 'I don't exactly remember it that way.' She gave me an example of her mother. Her mother had a very fast menopause. Ten minutes and it was over [laughter] . . . When we first got pregnant, my sister and I . . . she also said, 'No problems! None of us ever had any problems. You will be alright.'

Confidence was not merely the result of ignorance, however. The common theme across these accounts is that mothers 'got through' menopause. Even those who had listened in on adult conversations about serious health problems their mothers had suffered still felt confident. One woman said 'I sort of remember my mother going through it . . . I can remember her talking to her mother about flooding. I was never supposed to hear anything about it and I thought Ooh.' Her own confidence was unshaken: 'I'm hoping I just sail through it happily.'

These accounts are strikingly consistent in portraying menopause not as a transition but as a passage you come through. The mothers' menopause had not been seen (at least by these daughters) as an event, and irrevocable changes were not observed.

Daughters were thus encouraged to expect not a big change but a brief break in normal life:

> I am tending to think that it's a normal thing, that it will pass, that I'll come through it at the other end, if I do nothing, probably no worse off than anybody else. And, I look at my mother, and she's led a remarkably active life. I mean, she still plays sport, she's on the CAB, she runs around like a hairy-arse fly, and she's had no side-effects that I can see, so why should I? I asked my mother. I said, 'Did you experience flushes or did you find it difficult going through menopause?' She said, 'Look dear, I was so busy, I don't remember.'

Transitions, by contrast, are memorable.

How common was the metaphor of 'getting through' menopause? Text search is a blunt instrument in qualitative research, as people rarely use the same word or words to express the idea you are looking for. But in this material, the ability of our computer program to search text established the dominance of the metaphor of 'going through' as a way of thinking about menopause. A text search for 'going through' or 'been through' showed that phrase occurring in our data 545 times. Over 500 are in the context of midlife or menopause. 'Come through', 'get through' and 'sail through' also occurred frequently, and other women talked about coming 'out the other side'. These images of the woman sailing or ploughing *through* emphasise her own agency. They are much more common than images of something just ending without her effort: 'I'll be glad when it is over'; or standing in her way: 'I'd like the whole thing to be over and done with. It's just holding me up.' Getting, going, coming, sailing 'through' is by far the most common imagery used by the women we interviewed in the context of menopause.

The metaphor of a passage was familiar to us from the popular literature on menopause. Sheehy entitled her book *The Silent Passage* (1993), drawing on the idea of rites of passage in anthropology. In an important contribution to the literature on transitions, Glaser and Strauss (1970) constructed a theory of 'status passage', exploring the properties of passages from one status to another (how undesirable, how inevitable, do you go through it alone?). Women's experiences clearly varied on these dimensions. However the image of a passage or tunnel, which sometimes has light at the end, does not imply transition. Getting through is an achievement, you may be affected by it, scratched from the brambles you've bashed through, or muddy from the mire you've waded through. But whether you are *changed* when you are through — whether this is a transition — is quite a different question.

THE END OF SOMETHING

For some women, by contrast, menopause did signify the end of one stage of life, and the beginning of another. This was more likely to be due to social rather than physical changes, and it was in no case simply due to the one physical change defining menopause, the cessation of menses. Changes associated with a feeling that a stage had ended were related to ageing but not particularly menopause (e.g. wrinkles), or arguably associated with both (memory problems), or more generally with life stage (children leaving home), or career stage (promotion 'ceilings').

For a while we unquestioningly accepted the implication in the literature and in many of the group information sessions that all women experience this set of changes and that they add up to an over-all transition. However the data clearly showed that the changes were scattered over the years and rarely experienced as a set. Demographic data would indicate this, even if observation had not. Women in the 45–55 age group in our sample had children whose ages ranged from preschool to adult, only a minority were experiencing or even thinking about the 'empty nest' transition of children leaving home. As their workforce experience ranged from none to uninterrupted career building, retirement seldom featured. There was no set of changes always occurring together.

NO MORE PERIODS!

Of all these changes, the defining change of menopause, cessation of menses, was the least likely to be seen as a major transition and least likely to be regretted. For many women it was experienced not as an event but as an ambiguous and long process. It was frequently welcomed. Those who regretted it did not see it as a change in their identity. The only people to suggest this were advisers in group information sessions, who in several cases asserted that women were regarded as worthless once they could no longer reproduce. In one group session the organiser won a laugh telling the women that in society's view (in regard to menopause) 'What has happened is that you have out-lived your eggs and out-lived your usefulness.'

Our data disagree — cessation of menses is not usually a clear transition. It rarely marks an event: you never know when your periods have stopped. Irregularity of periods was often a major problem, women who suffered from it always looked forward to their cessation. 'Becoming so irregular and carting pads with you every day of your life became such an absolute bore.' However they were always unsure when it had happened:

> I would like my period to stop for good, instead of all the stopping and starting it is doing at present. I now go three or five months without one and then it will come for two months, regular twenty-eight days. I was always regular until five and a half years ago.

This woman's experience was of continuing uncertainty. 'Doctors say that it is the Change and you have to put up with it.'

Only women who had had a hysterectomy or sterilisation could specify a particular time of cessation of menses. This had caused a severe shock and feeling of loss for several at the time, but was now often a long-gone experience. Most other women had made determined and successful efforts to cease reproduction years before menopause, and we spoke with no woman for whom menopause had thwarted the intention to have a child. A very few, like Mary (see chapter 6), spoke of a sense of loss of fecundity, as part of the sense of growing old.

When a woman starts menstruating is a clear event that changes her irrevocably; in interviews many women recalled this time as a status passage. A few had been helped to celebrate it, most had found it confusing and learned it was taboo, but nobody had wondered whether or when something had changed.

BECOMING OLD

If cessation of menses is ambiguous and continuous, ageing is more so. It figures seldom in the data as a specific answer to the questions about change, but the open-ended interviews are full of fear of ageing. None of the women described menopause as a trigger for ageing, a view promoted by books encouraging women to take hormone replacement. However menopause was seen by the women we spoke to as a sign of ageing. As we will show in chapter 7, women thought others made that link. If it were known they were menopausal, they would suffer from the stereotype of the menopausal woman as unattractive and lacking in energy. The link of menopause with ageing occurs in most of the chapters in this book.

Becoming old is rarely seen as a clear transition. Only one set of comments suggests otherwise. When women 'saw' themselves as becoming what their mothers had become, it was in several cases reported as a discovery. In one health centre course we observed, a woman said the biggest shock she got was when she looked in the mirror one day and she could 'actually see' her mother. A few women remarked on similarity to their mothers, always with fear. These seemed to be comments about *becoming your mother* — and they were always negative:

> I notice that I've got my mother's hands . . . In the last eighteen months. I knew I was getting my mother's right hand about ten years ago.
>
> One profile I look and think, 'God it's Mum.'
>
> That happened this morning when I was having a shower with the shower cap on, and I thought, 'Oh, my mother.'
>
> Well, I usually see my mother when I look in the mirror and that's quite frightening, because it's my aged mother, or my middle-aged to older mother. And, that's quite painful. Because, it is not how I see myself.

THE BODY OUT OF CONTROL

More common than a sense of sudden ageing was a sense of loss of control over the body. Chapter 4 told some of the stories of women who felt their bodies had 'taken over', with unpredictable and unpleasant physical and psychological changes. These were always a shock, and women often recognised later that changes that had depressed or worried them were now under-standable as a pattern. The physical responses of their bodies had seemed to betray them, fail them, they were unable to read familiar body cues. But while these were often stressful experiences, they were never seen as signs of permanent body states:

> When I look back over perhaps a few years ago when I was really very touchy and uptight, I'm not sure whether it was because I was overworked or maybe it was the fact that the change of life was starting and I wasn't able to recognise it because I didn't know and I had nothing to go on.

Looking back, an elderly lady recalled the humiliation of a body out of control, but used the same phrase as many older women, 'I've been through all that':

> Trying to behave as if everything is normal, talking to a bank teller on a freezing day with the perspiration rolling down your face. And he looks at you as if you're half demented. I've been through all that. But, you know, somewhere at the end of the rainbow, you'll find you are back to normal again, and then you just feel sorry for women that you see going through it.

She was keen to let younger women know they would look back this way — but of course neither they nor we know if they will:

> I just think it's good to have the positive and negative signs, and have somebody there who has been through it, so that they know there is light at the end of the tunnel. It will all pass away, and life will be easy . . . Those going through it have got to have some hope.

One health adviser provided an insight into the processes that led women to interpret physical change as irrevocable transition. Her list of symptoms of menopause included 'hot flushes, dry vagina, loss of concentration, confusion, feeling worthless, loss of self esteem, aching joints, insomnia, irritability, looking old, feel life ends.'

The one exception to this was concern at loss of sexual drive. Women assumed that changes in their sexuality were permanent even when they assumed just as confidently that hot flushes would go away. Sometimes the two were linked, but they could laugh only at the hot flushes. One woman told us that her husband's way of supporting her through bad night sweats was to wear a full track-suit and socks, so she could turn the heat down on their water bed. When the flushes are troubling, 'He doesn't make any demands on me' but when she has 'a good day', 'You say, all right, it's your turn now, so come.'

EMPTY NEST

Each of the physical changes explored above was ambiguous, none of them clearly denoting transition. The same is true of social changes. These were mainly about family, experienced by women for whom family and home-making had been central.

Certainly for some women the 'empty nest' experienced when children left home was a very significant transition. Traditionally women's lives lose purpose when children leave home, and a few traditional women felt this. Our clearest account of a sharp alteration in family life came from a very elderly woman:

> Well, I think if a woman has been happily married, bearing children, and bringing the children up, and she has done that job . . . It is something you just are going to have to accept. It is a period of your life, one part of your life finishes and another part starts . . . Yes, feel positive about it, there is nothing you can do about it, it's a fact of life.

Like the loss of fecundity, the empty nest is a transition featuring more clearly in our data from community-level health advisers than in what women said to us. Both information leaflets and sessions bundled menopause into a package deal with changing family and 'empty nest'. Notes from one of the information sessions attended by members of our team record the adviser's messages:

The nurse said ... There are three areas of life. We should be looking forward to the last one at this stage. There was the young adolescence and then the years of pregnancy and bringing up a family. This often affects our attitude to life and we need to become far more positive... Menopause shouldn't be an awful time in life. It should be a looking-forward-to time.

In a telephone interview, a young community health nurse showed how these issues could be lumped together. The interviewer recorded:

> She said that menopause and midlife were one and the same and that women in their thirties may be incorporated. Midlife encompassed other areas such as life stage, empty nest. One of the most common symptoms was hot flushes. The aim at the centre was to offer other ways of dealing with menopause, not just medical.

A woman doctor made the point that children can leave home at other stages:

> People start to often look at these questions of who they are and what their meaning is as their own children grow up and start to leave. So, a woman may become depressed, it seems to me, when her oldest child suddenly goes away to boarding school at the age of 12 ... And they look at old people, and they look at old people's homes, and they look at their relationship with their husband, and they look at whether they've got a job, or if they haven't got a job. And, they can feel suddenly that they've got nothing, or what they've got is very drab, meaningless.

The well-documented double load of women caring for elderly and younger family members featured in some of these accounts:

> There's problems you know both sides with the generations, and you're ... the worm in the middle! ... with children who are bringing their problems, as they're growing up they're bigger problems than small children have, there isn't any doubt, and parents who are getting elderly ... I mean everybody gets their turn at it. We're there now.

All of these messages are depressing, and all certainly described the experiences of some women. It seemed more common, however, for women to expect, but not find, distress at the change:

> My children leaving home! I used to think it was going to be dreadful

when they have gone and two of them have gone . . . a couple of years, well, I sort of feel a sense of relief. Because, I suddenly realised that I am free to a degree. I still have a teenage daughter at home but I am free from two of them. I was really locked into the house or looking after them, whereas now I think about myself more and I suddenly think, 'Hey I have a bit of freedom!'

For a few women, this new freedom was an extraordinary arrival at a new stage of life — a clear transition that was extremely positive:

> I would say free. Not from a menopausal point of view but I would say free in the fact that I have got employment where I can do to a large extent a lot of things as I want to and when I want to. I have control of that. For the last twenty years I've had kids. You can't go on holidays or you can but you have to think about kids and animals and all these sorts of things. The animals one by one have all dropped dead. The children, it doesn't matter whether they are at home or not, they're independent and are quite capable of standing on their own two feet. They can cook and do everything for themselves. They don't need me. Which means for the first time in my life I can do as I please.

AVOIDING TRANSITION

Inevitably, HRT is a character in this drama. It appears in the comparisons of women's lives now and 'then'; a promise of a way of avoiding change, of just going on as you were. The theme intruded in a group discussion of memories of mothers:

> It must have been terrible for our mothers to experience all these symptoms and really have nothing to take to relieve it.

> I can remember my mother sort of getting hot and bothered and cranky and when I look back I used to think, 'Gosh, my mother was bad tempered.' Now I think, 'That poor woman!' She suffered the same sort of symptoms that I suffer, she couldn't talk about it and she had nothing. I really feel very sorry for her and very disgusted.

In this context the HRT promise will be easily accepted:

> My mother — and I have got to go back — went through the most horrendous menopause you could ever imagine. And I thought there is no way that I would put anybody through what she went through . . .

> in my mother's day I think ignorance was bliss and people . . . from the medical profession to families had no knowledge so really tended to avoid it . . . I decided that I would do something about it, I don't want as I said before to go through what my mother went through.

Interestingly, all the women who recalled their mothers' having trouble were determined to use modern medical science to avoid this.

Women's literature has for years beamed messages to women that they should avoid taking a medical way through a social transition. During our study several very influential, and heavily publicised, books appeared, but, as shown in chapter 3, they were balanced by a bulk of popular literature presenting the promise of HRT and debating its risks. As earlier chapters showed, women in our study had almost always heard the promise of HRT and rarely accepted it without concern.

In chapter 9 we return to the issues of medical advice and women's interpretations of it. In the present context, one aspect of that complex relationship of doctors' knowledge and power is particularly relevant. When women resisted medical advice to take HRT, they almost always felt the doctor was making false promises that it would help them avoid transition. A woman dealing with very serious family problems had sought advice for depression and been given HRT:

> I went out with a prescription in my hand and came home and thought, 'This isn't fair you know, it's sort of blaming me, but it really isn't my problem.' 'It's causing me worry, but it wasn't caused by ME', and it just seemed to me like too easy an answer, that I was sort of being wiped off, as really, 'You're the problem! If we put you on medication then the rest of the family all fall into place.' And I must admit I really didn't like the answer.

In her wording, agency is denied. Even women who researched and made a decision about HRT tended to talk about the doctor 'putting me on it'. The imagery is absurd; it implies that, like a doll put on a shelf, she can only stay on it. A text search in QSR NUD•IST for 'put me on/her on' found these words used ninety-two times! But while few claimed agency for having decided on HRT, many intended to use it for long-term prevention of change.

Transition work

We were startled by the range of fatalism but also the range of agency. No women merely received change. Some women welcomed and some accepted it, some saw their lives as proceeding uninterrupted. For some, changes seemed to build cumulatively, triggering further changes, one change igniting another for a seemingly endless series of explosions. We have many accounts of general optimism, like this celebration of something much less than transition, but more than resignation:

> I just think that around the age of 40, a lot of women see new needs in their lives. I don't know if it happens to everybody, but it certainly has happened to me. And it has happened to a lot of women I've spoken to. Some women never change. But others are looking for something new in their lives, and new things start happening to them.

A few were different because they sought control of both private and public aspects of their lives at this stage, and some achieved it. Their stories are triumphant, but uncommon. In all this data, we heard six stories of what I termed 'transition work', processes of working at making and managing transition, taking charge of the direction of change and taking advantage of the opportunity to effect it. To understand these processes requires an approach to transitions not often found in the literature, in which people are seen as agents, not merely recipients of change.[1]

Many questions cannot be answered by our data. When are women most likely to manage transitions, when are they more likely to be victims? What contexts and factors make it easier? What are the sources of help in transition work? Which women are able to achieve this control? We have too few examples to generalise. We do know that the women we talked to saw the ability to take control of menopause as a modern phenomenon, and that they linked this to the health-promotion theme explored in chapter 10: taking responsibility for your health. In all this data, no women talked of their mothers doing transition work. Wise or foolish, long-suffering or lucky, the women of the older generation were portrayed as victims of their bodily change:

I don't believe in genes because I think I was completely different to my mum. My mum didn't exercise whereas I think if you get out and keep your parts moving and everything, you are helping yourself.

With so few cases, patterns can't be explored. However the idea of transition work can be illustrated by one woman's story. It was striking that the women who most clearly took charge of their lives during the intermission of menopause did it solo.

Jay had a hysterectomy ten years ago. She recalls with pleasure and almost vindictive delight the control she took at that time over her life, her work, and her marriage. After recently experiencing dramatic menopausal 'symptoms', she took sick leave. She is about to return to work from this second experience of what she terms 'time out'. The first opportunity was provided by surgery:

> Before I went in people said 'Oh you will be sick, so and so had [a hysterectomy] and she has never been well' and I thought , 'Oh well there's no point in worrying about it'. I wasn't going to have a period any more and to me it was wonderful because I had had period pains for thirty years . . . Anyway I had the hysterectomy and I was told not to do anything and for the first time in my life I did nothing. And I sat and stared out a window, once I got home, and I really didn't do anything. And I am a very active person! I really went over my life and worked it all out.

A colleague at work had died, and the loss had 'gone right down deep':

> I worked all through that. My relationship with my husband, everything. I just sat. I read *War and Peace* and stared out of the window. That is what I did for about eight weeks and then I went back to work and have never looked back.

Later she explains that having to take time out 'gave me a chance to work on my brain'. Controlling the body was part of this process:

> The only positive thing about me having periods was [that] I had five healthy children and I never really had any trouble having children. I was always sick with pregnancies but only morning sickness. I never had anything wrong medically. Everything worked the way it was supposed to work.

Jay digresses to an account of an accidental pregnancy; the common theme is control. The transcript conveys the delight in control, as well as in doing the socially undesirable, rejecting women's duties, just sitting and, in odd contrast to this passivity, taking charge:

> I didn't know what to do and I was panic stricken; when I had the abortion relief was the only thing I felt. And that was how I felt after the hysterectomy. I didn't even think about losing womanhood or anything like that it was just relief. No more periods. No more pain... I had been someone who had chopped all the wood for the house, I did all the housework, the gardening and I physically did everything that had to be done. I milked goats, I bred poultry, I did my own gardening and so I had led a very physical life that went from 5 a.m. to 11 p.m. ... So when I was told to sit, I just sat. Just for once I was going to sit and I realised I needed that time.

'Time out' is a recurring phrase. What happens in time out? In basketball, it is the special chance, the seconds ticking, a tiny interval in which strategy can be switched, the team drawn together. Use the time well, don't hesitate, take charge, redirect. When the teams run back on after time out, the game can be totally changed, the expectations of the audience confounded. After the hysterectomy, Jay had 'no pains, no anything':

> It was wonderful. I was free for the first time. No periods, every twenty-eight days for five full days — it was just wonderful. Physically it has been wonderful ever since and I think probably looking back that is when I started working out my life and who I am and what I am and my relationships with other people. I started giving my poor husband a hard time but he has gone along with it . . . I think I have put everything on hold.

An interesting phrase. What is it to put things on hold? A telephonist puts you on hold, making you wait till it suits her to attend to your request. That allows efficient management of multiple demands, and perhaps a wicked sense of power.

The medical profession contributed little. Jay had gone to a female doctor two years earlier:

> I thought I was going through menopause then because I was bursting into tears a lot and I was very forgetful and depressed and they were

a bit rough to me down there. One woman gave me an internal and said I was far too young and don't be ridiculous . . . I went to . . . an endocrinologist. Anyway he thought that I might have been but he wasn't sure so he put me on — he gave me oestrogen.

It's interesting that Jay corrects the phrase implying lack of agency, 'he put me on'. Her next decision was to take herself off HRT, after two weeks. 'I had such pains in the head and legs I stopped that and thought I would work it out for myself.' Working it out involved departing from mainstream medical advice, another episode of control:

> I started on vitamins and minerals and vitamin E and stuff like that. It sort of settled down and I started this course of study and I didn't have time to think about those sorts of things so I put all that on hold because I was studying such long hours and didn't have time for any illness at all.

The same concentration on time, and that phrase again, 'putting things on hold', deciding, taking charge. At the same time Jay was starting a part-time course, and meeting physical and psychological changes, including hot flushes:

> I started getting very short — and I hated my husband and I resented him . . . I would be so agitated and then I thought, I thought it is not menopause, it is something else. I wasn't depressed and I was taking calcium and vitamin E, vitamin B because I don't eat meat . . . I have been home for seven weeks and in that time those palpitations have gone and I really actively worked through why I was resenting people. I have been reading books on anger, communication, assertiveness, you know personal relationships and things like that and I have been inclined to work through it all and I feel I have now worked through my relationship with my husband.

Work, family and the body are intricately interwoven in the story. Jay finds it hard to disentangle their contributions to her distress or its solution:

> I used to worry a lot about [work relations] and I wasn't sure and then I think also I was working through my relationship with my husband. The children were older and instead of focusing on the children which I had done for years I switched the focus to me . . . I did do a little thinking at the beginning of the holiday. Either Sire and

I would end up divorced or I would have thought this situation out. This resentment was what I had to work on but it was really me I was working on not so much him.

In both of the stages where a break has been grasped, the opportunity was provided by physical, gynaecological problems, and much of the solution was in solitary physical work. Jay calls herself 'a very physical person':

> Whilst I didn't actually sit this time and stare into space, I was gardening or digging and I remember my brain was working the whole time and then I was reading these books and trying to work through things and so I would think . . . Often somebody would be talking to me . . . but I would be switched off. They would ask if I was alright and I said, 'Yes I am just working through, but I will be alright.' Or I would be outside in the garden digging and that is wonderful. The brain works and oh I love that. I am up and down the hill with the wheelbarrow 'cause it is hard work at our place. My brain worked the whole time. I work in the rain as well so I am left on my own, they call me Paddington Bear.

Menopause was both central and peripheral; almost as a stranger Jay monitors her body and reports on it.

> I remember thinking, 'I seem to have ovulating pains,' and I remember it sort of passing through my mind, 'I wonder if this is a last dance from my body' . . . I found the hot flushes weakening, really weakening, because I couldn't get a decent night's sleep. I kept waking up. I have been taking Primrose oil. I have doubled the dosage and touch wood it is much better. I am sleeping right through at night now.

While Jay is aware of working at achieving these changes, she has no clear picture of the ways that she has taken control. 'I can't explain how I feel better but I do. I can tackle the world.' She will now happily advise others, especially women facing hysterectomy:

> I always tell them, 'Enjoy it. Make the best of it.' You get rid of something you don't need . . . I always say 'sit for eight weeks and enjoy it because you will never get a legitimate opportunity like this again and take full advantage of it'.

This advice is followed, as though linked to it, by a happy account of a much more recent domestic episode:

> I stayed in bed the other day and read *The Power of One* all day. I stopped reading at one a.m. and I had started at nine in the morning. It was lovely. I kept laughing to myself and thinking this is wonderful and I kept reading and would get up and get another cup of tea. And even yesterday Sire came home in the afternoon. I'd been up all morning, I had washed up and cleaned up all the things I usually do and went back to bed with my book. He came in about four [p.m.] and said 'Oh you are having a lovely time aren't you!' and I said, 'Yes just wonderful!' 'Do you want a cup of tea?' 'Yes please' [laughter].

In all this assessing, interpreting, resolving, she has been alone. She chooses not to talk to other women, constrained, as so many are, by her social context and particularly by the workplace and women's place in it:

> JAY: I think I have been a bit wary . . . Somehow I have this fear that it would be used against me . . . I really have no grounds for thinking that other than perhaps people that I have heard in the past say 'Oh she is going through the Change.' So I guess I was really wary of that . . . This is the most I think I have ever talked.
> LYN: I think that is probably true of most of us.

MENOPAUSE RESEARCH AS A HEALTH HAZARD

When I was first asked, as a qualitative methodologist and family sociologist, to join in an application for the grant on menopause, I refused, on the grounds that I had no interest in the subject and that if I did, it would get me! I was 46, and over the next years it did. I approached the project fascinated by the methodological challenge, but in complete ignorance of the topic (my previous books were all on the early stages of marriage and family and I thought HRT stood for the computer terminology of 'hard carriage return'). My first hot flushes hit on my forty-seventh birthday. During the following year I anticipated and recognised each tiny body change through the project's data. For me, and some of the other women on the project, the experience was of having a transition constructed for us. My concern grew that education campaigns would put other women in the same position, fostering awareness of heaps of 'symptoms' that cumulatively created a sense of irrevocable change. The following section is from a memo written in June 1992:

> I have noticed my own tendency to link known symptoms and see them as sets. The fingernails breaking would not have mattered had I not suspected this too was a symptom of menopause, and that it further indicated loss of calcium or skin strength or both. And this brings on the whole package of fears, now *known* as a package — osteoporosis, heart attack, the lot. A package deal. Interesting how hard it is for me not to see it as such, even though I now have enough data to be sure of the variety of experience. I don't have data showing that other women feel this way, but somehow feel they must. Dangerous stuff this — terribly important not to project my own very unusual research-led experience of menopause onto the data.
>
> What *do* I have? A lot of speculation. Given the publicity to especially osteoporosis, there is an image of menopause now, a public stereotype. For all the assertions about unfortunate images in the past, the women seem to say that there was no such image — only a gentle, regretful feeling that something had gradually drawn to an end. Now we are being told about grim reapers, loss of sexuality, and an event, a point at which there is a treatment to be applied for known dangers. If it's not danger of hip fracture and heart attack, it's danger of cancer from HRT. I increasingly feel we must speak to older women, to find if this is new, the assertion of a sharp-edged chasm in women's lives, no mere bridge from one biological stage to another.
>
> On this argument, women are not necessarily benefited by the community-level determined education campaigns. My own experience suggests it is not a help to know of all the awful things that can happen; an image is built by lectures on stress incontinence and brittle bones, and Amanda's and Maureen's reports of the groups confirm the liturgy of negative themes in them. I am now in that age group — dare I laugh or climb a mountain for fear of peeing in my pants or breaking a hip (respectively)? It is not a help to know that loss of libido and sexual difficulties, vaginal horrors and atrophy are confidently anticipated — a sense of defiance as I think of sex, anxiety at the slightest itch. It does not help at all to be classified by an age cohort — not something that has happened to me before, and it should not have happened now.
>
> Of course, it helps to know what's happening to you and know what can be done. That's the thesis of empowerment. But power to do what? Recognise that you can survive it by talking to women with awfuller symptoms than yours, doing t'ai chi and laughing about hot

flushes — that all makes perfectly good sense. Except that seeing and knowing those symptoms as a set creates problems of its own.

What other life stage is prepared for in this way? Puberty is approached by excitement and warnings (how not to get pregnant), not lectures on pre-menstrual syndrome and acne. Pregnancy and birthing classes don't go into the details of everything that can go wrong and the medical answers — nobody would continue to full-term if they did! At the community level, women are not herded into information nights to learn of breech births and how to deal with a deformed child. The difference? No single 'cure' for those is the obvious answer, but I think it's too obvious. Many of the women running community-level stuff are opposed to HRT or worried about it and wanting to 'validate' women's experience as positive and/or available for public discussion. Difference is that they too see it as an entirely negative time and a transition into danger.

Seeing the symptoms as a set means that women experiencing just one mildly will then start looking for the lot. Cathi Lewis charged into the research office saying 'It's got me: I had hot flushes!! It's this bloody project!' I recognised my dry mouth as a 'symptom' when I reviewed a manuscript. The public health case is for Cathi and me to know that's a symptom of menopause so we won't worry about it. But stuff that — I'd have assumed I was just dry from central heating or a slight cold or major stress. I'd much rather just be not interested in dry throats, and take a glass of water to lectures, than see this as yet another one of the symptoms in the set . . .

The feminist response is to approach midlife proudly, looking forward to the next stage, rustling up a bit of zest, denying the need to be 'young' and attractive as defined in a youth-oriented society. That is, I think, probably a grave simplification, and as a card-carrying feminist I'm having trouble with it. Even if you don't enjoy being young and attractive, there are manifest advantages in it for all sorts of more acceptable goals like authority. The stereotype of the transition involves not just dry skin and thinning hair but also mood swings, memory loss and the fear of being incompetent and a 'little old lady'. I'm sure that I have for years repeated myself, forgotten names and lost my keys (that dates from parenthood) with chaotic results. But since the first hot flush, hearing myself repeat a story, or goof a name or stress out when the keys aren't on the fridge has new, dire, implications. There's fear there, because these are the NEXT stage after midlife — and I do not want to be there. Nor do I want to be unattractive to men, to myself or to the world at large. Like Carmel's interviewee, I enjoy being able to summon attention, and enjoy being able to effect my own ends — and I know that will be less easy when I'm less attractive . . .

We have, in our different ways, stumbled on an ethically problematical topic for women researchers . . . In asking about menopause we contribute to processes by which women are forced to redefine themselves at the arrival of any experience socially defined to include health risk. We are doing it to ourselves: first I, then Cathi, having clear symptoms after the project began. OK, that's not a statistically significant result, and we both bit the topic because we felt involved in the issue (we'll worry about the research-generated menopause when Nicole has her first hot flush!). But we both have said similar things, laughingly, about recognition of other symptoms. Do we do it to other women? Should we? Do they want us to? Should we interpret their eagerness to talk as indicating approval? All the issues of ethics of qualitative research are here.

I am writing this chapter four years after that memo. This year, my children both moved away from home, my mother survived a heart attack, and I resigned from my tenured academic position of twenty-six years to work full-time in a new career of research software development. No hot flushes though!

New Transitions?

Our data show no women eagerly anticipating menopause. The messages they hear are about physical debilitation, declining energy and attractiveness. The impact of these messages is more dramatic because these women, born postwar, were the first cohort to have adult lives not predetermined by the traditional line-up of socially required major transitions: leaving home, marrying, having children. They blurred the transitions that had been so clear for their mothers (child/adult, single/married, childless/parent, work/home). Their adult lives could be led independent of fathers and husbands, and careers in the paid workforce were quite normally continued after marriage and even after childbearing. They came to adulthood as the second wave of feminism challenged traditional family values and patriarchal public life. Many won workforce participation and career advancement only after child-rearing, and many felt it had been a hard fight.

As these women reached midlife, the new public debate on menopause began. The Change had been newly defined, by an odd coalition of medical authority and feminist critique, as a major transition for all women, always unwelcome, at worst to be dreaded, at best accepted with resignation or with determination. With a new 'cure' in HRT, it was also defined as an avoidable change.

Not all women expect or experience a marked change at this time. If they do, not all experience physical symptoms or personal crises that deserve distress. For a lot of women, menopause is, as one put it, 'no big deal'. For some, the social definition of menopause is the main problem; they are told to expect change and to be distressed, and people around them label them with that expectation.

There is a plethora of literature on transition. Most of it proved of limited use to us. It treats transitions as events, not processes, and people as recipients rather than participants, victims of change rather than actors who make it. Certainly some transitions look like events that happen to people, largely beyond their control or construction (such as starting school, being sacked or death), but even these are better understood as passages, from one state to another, and menopause, for most of the women we talked with, was not. Nor did they normally merely *receive* a transition. They differed greatly in their interest in actively rethinking and remaking their lives, and their ability to do so. While few women reported the sort of dedicated work at transition that Jay had achieved, throughout this data there is a strong sense of women participating in the *making* of their changes. They showed us a very great range of what I have termed 'transition work': the processes of preparing for, anticipating, interpreting and controlling the outcomes of transition. The next chapter tells one such story, through a woman's diary.

6
ONE WOMAN'S STORY

Mary Fisher

Informed intuition, rather than navel gazing, is generally a guiding principle of my life. Thus it was with slight misgiving I volunteered to keep this journal for a year. Would it become a self-fulfilling prophesy? Would I wallow in a morass of imagined symptoms? How could my meanderings be of any relevance to other women (and men)? I had asked my very religious mother about the onset and duration of her menopause. I thought the information might be useful to her six daughters — I'm the eldest. Her response: 'When it happens, it happens. It's God's law.' For my vicarious daughters and sisters here is one person's version of 'what happens'.

Sunday, 9 August 1992
Tonight in the image vein, I'm mourning the loss of me — the energetic, bright, articulate and alert whirling dynamo who has metamorphosed into a large slug. This new creature yearns for time to rest, reflect and re-energise. There's a picture of lilies in my kitchen — a constant reminder of my basic philosophy. Consider the lilies of the field. They neither toil nor spin. The orthodox religious tag that completes the above quote is not important to me. But the message is. When I die I'd like just one white lily on my coffin. A symbol of my lucky life. I'm not afraid of death.

What a maudlin first entry ... Stiffen the spine and talk of symptoms. Hurl off blankets at 1.05 a.m. and 4.05 a.m. most days. However, the hot flushes seem to be diminishing in intensity, frequency and duration. Maybe because it's winter. I'm not disciplined enough to make a proper survey of the times, etc. Other resented signs of this ageing process? Drying skin, toenails becoming harder and hornier, to say nothing of two recalcitrant hairs that keep popping out on cheek and chin every other day. They require a razor. I have little grey hair — I think that's genetic.

Internal processes show signs of wear. I think I am forgetful. I have always written messages on my hand — I lose pieces of paper at a rate of knots. It's disconcerting to be standing in a supermarket staring at one's palm trying to decode the abbreviations that form the shopping list — written but half an hour previously. The body joints creak each morning. It was cheering to hear a young Olympian complain of the same, even if the reasons were different.

Monday, 17 August 1992
Random thoughts. I've never been a person who gets really ill. I've never had malaria even though I lived in a highly malarial area for six years (in the sixties). All around me people disappear for two weeks with virulent doses of the latest virus. I don't get sick enough to take any time off. I'd love to spend two weeks in bed free of any responsibilities. However, I'd probably get bored. At this stage of my life I seem to be reacting much more to all kinds of external stimuli — house dust, perfumes, soaps etc. My eyes get sore and I don't always bother with eye make-up.

Sunday, 23 August 1992
I have rarely bought new things preferring the notion of recycling. I've also had a kind of policy of not having matching objects in my home. It's a reaction against economic rationalism, consumerism and yuppiedom. I'm quite happy to be considered eccentric. If I'd had children it might have been different. I think youthful peer pressure has a spin-off effect upon parents. Anyhow at this stage

of my life I find myself buying brand new furniture and not having to justify the purchases.

Wednesday, 2 September 1992
Spring and the garden. I visited a young friend in hospital with her second child. Walked up ten flights of stairs at the Women's Hospital. I'm remembering lots of things from childhood with a special affection. I don't know how my mother ever managed. (I am the eldest of twelve children.) I find myself so often behaving in ways that I can identify with her — 'my mother myself' stuff! I have a great deal more admiration for her. My Tasmanian sister, on her way home from an overseas trip, commented that Mum seems much more forgetful. I said that it doesn't matter because if she doesn't remember it doesn't really matter.

Germaine's book (*The Change*) sits on my pillow. I went to school with her and think her book is well researched. When I used to wake up in the middle of the night thinking I was dying, I'd grab her book, look up the relevant section via the index, and go back to sleep reassured. I don't need to do that anymore. I have a feeling that everything will be all right.

Sunday, 20 September 1992
Rose at seven — washed, cleaned mopped, gardened and checked the roof in an effort to beat the body into submission. It worked about 90%. Reflecting on the past few weeks I seem to crash on the weekend. Yet I look forward to weekends. In all my time at my present work, seventeen years, I have had only about four sick days off. I've lectured with roaring migraines and kept going in that tradition of Catholic guilt that was drummed into me as a child. God has a lot to answer for!

Sunday, 27 September 1992
I find I'm looking backwards a lot. Perhaps this is a concern for the coming generation — into which I have had no genetic input. In that backwards vein — I have always regarded Autumn, the season of my birth, as my favourite season. However, last week I changed.

Musing during one of the recent heavy rain storms, I decided that I like spring better. It will now be my favourite season. No matter what kind of a gale is blowing or how hard it is raining there are always signs of new life — embryonic buds on trees, rosebuds emerging from their lush new leaves and blazes of colour in every direction. So, bud on spring! A friend and I planted some seeds on Showday. I've always liked growing plants from seed, even though it takes longer for the final product. Another symbol of children.

Yesterday was my mother's seventy-third birthday. I took her out to lunch, and again noted all those similarities.

Saturday, 3 October 1992
Aching joints. Visitors arrive and tell me things I've done recently — for example, a birthday present of plants. I find that I can't even remember giving them, or when.

I'm a bit paranoid too. I'll have to work on that. I was asked by our Victorian Principal to go on a selection panel for heads of school and heads of department. I decided that I was asked as a kind of also-ran. It took all day Friday and was a great learning experience. However I found I usually had to wait for others to give an opinion before I was confident enough to voice mine — which usually tallied with theirs, or even illuminated their opinion. Sometimes, quite often, I feel like Chauncy, the character in *Being There*. That was the film of the book in which a colander head became president of the United States. I feel like that. If a flap was lifted on my head there'd be a colander inside the head of this apparently successful woman.

Friday, 9 October 1992
I've had many meetings during the week. As a result I've decided that it's a very male-dominated world. I'm not a feminist by persuasion, more of an equalist. However, I've been listening keenly all week to male-dominated language and values. There is no place in their world for menopausal women — not that that topic was ever raised or alluded to — it's just my conclusion from what appears to be their view of the world.

Friday, 16 October 1992
I HATE growing old, being old, being anywhere. Everything is Bosch. This term applies to days when no good feature — of the day or other people — can be seen. It's as if Hieronymus himself has painted the day with his allegorical figures. If I cannot see/perceive even a well-formed nose, kindly eyes, well-kept shiny hair, an attractive personality, a hint of inner strength or anything positive about my fellow humans, then it is a Bosch day indeed. It's been a bit like that for the past week. I have painted myself slater grey and just want to crawl under the nearest cool log or rock and stay there permanently. I want to sleep a whole night through — not wander aimlessly around the house and back garden trying to cool off at 3 a.m. I want to be cool — in more ways than one! I'd like to be tiny. I sometimes think that one day I'll just explode into the stratosphere and all my bits will be forever dissipated.

Tuesday, 20 October 1992
I've been thinking a great deal about what I mean about being more reflective — looking backwards instead of forwards. I've never reflected much on the past, except perhaps to learn from my mistakes. But now images of the past are being triggered off by a range of events/items. The corner of a picture, the flash of a particular colour, a face, a drift of perfume or an aroma can trigger a flood of memories from childhood or later. Happy memories, not sad ones. I guess it's all to do with not wanting to face the reality of old age. All this hormonal activity just to give birth to old age.

Monday, 26 October 1992
I was particularly taken with an article in the weekend *Australian Magazine* about Fred Hollows. He quoted lines from Emerson:

> To leave the world a bit better,
> Whether by a healthy child or a garden patch
> Or a redeemed social condition,
> To know even one life has breathed easier
> Because you lived,
> This is to have succeeded.

Grandiose sentiments in a way, and all the more contradictory when I tell you that I went to the doctor today and asked for a week off. Not for any physical illness — just general I don't want to go on anymore, or to do anything. She reminded me that my life was fairly full of looking after others. I reminded her that that was because I am such a compulsive person. Not many people understand that. I am finding it difficult to organise myself when I am left to my own devices. I think this is a kind of warning. I have to be for myself before I can really be for others. So here I am at home with a week off. It will take me several days to cope with the guilt of not being at work. However, I shall fight it.

Saturday, 28 November 1992
It's almost midnight and I've just gone through several hours of being angry. Why? Each weekend I feel I should do uni work and in fact every day of the week there is work work to be done at home. At present I have about a hundred assignments to correct. and an evaluation to process. However, I decided to have Saturday off. It didn't work. By teatime I had a head full of guilt and ache. So, even though I watched a program on TV, here I am having spent three hours on work work. I'm sick of it. Maybe I'm just inefficient. It would be so nice to come home and be a happy vegetable, or to spend time pottering on the roof or weeding the garden, or rearranging the house or sewing or whatever. I am tired of being haunted by piles of paper begging me, haunting me to interact with them.

During 1992 I have had only about four days leave. Moan, moan! It's my own fault. I had two weeks leave scheduled for before Christmas but they have just gone up in smoke in a slew of meetings. I should concentrate on giving birth to my independence. On the other hand I am a creature well acquainted with discomfort anxiety. Give me something that has to be done, especially of the heavy academic variety and I will wash curtains, mop floors, sort through filing cabinets or just get under the doona to delay the start of the task.

I'd like to be able to write. I've decided that I'm a person with a fear of closure. Now that was okay when I was able to juggle many things at once. A whirl of activity and busyness evoked sympathy. No wonder some things weren't finished. There were always so many to do. That excuse won't wash any more. I'm finding it really hard to change that pattern of behaviour. I feel that I'm always on a slippery surface over which I leave a trail of unfinished wreckage. At this stage of my life this trail is not embryonic and bursting with the promise of new ideas and insights. It's more reminiscent of a sweep of frowsy autumn litter. On the other hand this twelve months of journal is just a frozen-in-time snapshot of my life. I think I am attempting to widen the pictorial edges to give you a bigger canvas. It's also a way of saying I haven't always been like this. But all my worst habits seem to be exaggerated.

Friday, 4 December 1992
The Christmas month — full of women with Christmas-ham haunches and plum pudding bellies (including myself). It's been a particularly bloody week so I am being slightly venomous. It's also because I have a ditch-digger's physique. That's partly my genetic inheritance and the result of having dieted since I was about 16. Now, my body could survive on a lettuce leaf and I have great difficulty in accepting this large burden that I must kick-start into action every day. I'm *au fait* with a great deal of the literature about weight, diet, body type and the like and I've just given up. I have almost banned anyone from taking my photo. I do not want permanent evidence of myself in anyone's photo album. Better to remember the me that lives inside.

Tuesday, 8 December 1992
I am still out of sorts. I don't know where my sorts have gone to. Busy weekend. My niece had a twenty-first birthday. That meant a trip to Glen Waverley — the other end of the earth . . . My 47-year-old sister from Launceston had come over for the party. She thinks she is beginning menopause. We had a chat about it. I particularly mentioned that I'd been trying too hard to focus on

the childless notion. She agreed and said that she had absolutely no regrets that she hadn't had children.

Thursday, 10 December 1992
I am depressed, sick, hot, tired and my colander head is also in a fog. Ah woe! I have not laughed much. If anyone were to ask me a question, a question about anything at all, I would probably answer 'seven and a quarter' or 'nineteen' or any other number. My brain has gone into recession. Why is it so? There is too much to do. Perhaps I am reacting against having to cancel my leave. I have not corrected my other pile of forty essays. I am in a black tunnel. My body is hurting. The hot weather means that my inner thighs rub together, shred my panty hose and cause me discomfort. My long labia are drying out and rubbing together like scrunchy autumn leaves.

Tuesday, 15 December 1992
I am in full flow of a period, the first for more than a year. My body is shucking the last evidence of its fertility potential. It's official! I can now produce bum stickers that say 'It's not my fault. It's genetic.' A newspaper item explained recent research reported in a medical journal. A gene for overweight has perhaps been isolated. That is absolutely no consolation to me. My mother, who is built like an ox, tells of her Aunty May — died at 96 weighing 20 stone. She had had ten children. Another of her aunts was of similar weight. She lasted until she was 92. I don't think I want to carry this body burden around for that long.

Thursday, 24 December 1992
I am exhausted. I do not like Christmas. There is too much sadness and poverty around. I can see that I'll have to go in to work again in a few days.

Friday, 25 December 1992
Christmas night. It has been a good day. My immediate family of forty people had lunch together. A good family turn. Too much food

of course, but good company. It's great that one's family is always so accepting of one — warts, blemishes, excess kilos and all.

Tuesday, 29 December 1992
My neighbour's mother is here from Hong Kong. We had a great celebration with other neighbours, my mother and some of my sisters too. My neighbour Jane is from Swaziland. During the night my mother asked me about Jane's country of origin. I said 'Swaziland.'
Mum said, 'She's really dark isn't she?'
Me — 'She's from Africa, Mum.'
Mum follows the West Indians in the cricket and keeps saying. 'I do hope the Darkies win.' My mother was brought up with seven city cousins after her own mother died when Mum was 7. She has a fine intelligence which she chooses to keep hidden. Her only ambition was to have many children. Of my eleven siblings all but one have had tertiary education, mostly on scholarships. She has done a remarkable job.

Friday, 1 January 1993
So glad to see the end of '92. I think 1993 is a prime number. I didn't make any New Year's resolutions but then I don't usually. I'd like to just survive the present and then get my life sorted out. I have recognised that I'm a real hoarder. But I'm not really attached to possessions. They are just here for those who might need them.

Sunday, 10 January 1993
I had really nagging neck and back pain for a few days. Then I discovered a lump behind my left ear. I have never been a panic merchant as far as my health is concerned. I've always believed that any minor irritation would pass with no interference especially of the medical variety. I've divided my family into those with internal health problems and those with structural ones. I belong in the latter category. Backaches as a result of unloading planes in New Guinea, hurling bluestone around the backyard and moving

furniture with little regard for proper back alignment. (My mother still moves large items of furniture around when she thinks they'd look better in another position. She belongs in the structural category with her bung knee.) Now, however, I tend to panic a bit. I can understand how some nurses (I have a sister and a sister-in-law who are nurses) and doctors respond to children's ailments. My response is as follows (actually it's just a way of coping):

- head lump = brain tumour or galloping lymph glands
- joint ache= immediate replacement operation
- cut= gangrene
- one extraneous hair on face= all encompassing thatch
- anything else is bound to be cancer

I went to see the doctor and of course the lump was nothing and the growing spots on my upper back are incipient warts. I had a few items written in my diary to talk to Angela (my doctor) about. I couldn't decipher one that read 'b'out' — I'd only written it half an hour before. Angela thought it might stand for black out. 'No,' I said, 'I don't have them.'

'Well does it mean burn out?'

' Oh yes,' I said, 'I was wondering if you thought I might be a bit burnt out?'

'Burnt out,' she said, 'Incinerated and cremated as well.'

Thursday, 28 January 1993
One more day to go [until I return to work]. I am still not sleeping well. I am dreadfully tired all day but at night I sleep in small snatches, wander round the house trying to cool off and get up when I wake up quite early. I have had flushes all day and at night too. There is no point in wearing make-up which will just run off my face. My hair needs washing constantly because it quickly becomes damp and dank. Some of the skin on my face seems to be changing. My nose is breeding large pores. Yuk. I have to get stronger glasses — bifocals at that. I have had difficulty reading the subtitles on TV. I am long-sighted. I have never attracted biting

insects. Now they dare to venture close to or onto me. Is there any causality between skin temperature and insect attraction?

Thursday, 4 February 1993
There has been a cool change. I am beginning to feel more like myself — because of the weather and because I am on leave. At the same time I am discovering more bits that are going astray. I have a rash of warts behind my right knee. This has led me to muse about parts of one's anatomy that cannot readily be seen. I'd like to insert an indiarubber neck extension to myself. It could be of an Alice-through-the-looking-glass variety. Just nibble the corner of this loaf and your neck will be six feet long. Imagine the careful inspection that could be done. Small toenails — the ones on the end of each foot, could be cut with ease. The back could be examined at my leisure for bumps and skin irregularities.

Thursday, 11 March 1993
Another week. I wish I lived in a caravan like Milly Molly Mandy. (Note this reflection back to well-remembered childhood characters.) A caravan would be so much less fuss. Why this wish? I had to climb onto the roof to fix the TV aerial. My legs just will not obey me anymore. Nor the rest of my body. Fixing the aerial required perching on some ridge capping on part of the slate roof and undoing and redoing some wiring. Some time later, after I had slithered and slid to retrieve dropped objects and to retrieve myself from further down the roof, I had not succeeded in fixing the aerial. I had only succeeded in putting my feet right through six slates. I had to call a plumber to fix them.

Monday, 15 March 1993
Visitors came here for election night and Clothilde was also staying here experiencing her first Australian election. A surprising, but welcome result. I am feeling better but am very low on energy. I had to go to the doctor for a Pap smear. It was okay. The blood pressure was okay. Yippee.

Monday, 29 March 1993
Home from Hong Kong, a three-hour turn around and off to Perth — for work and to stay with my sister, her husband and three children. How wonderful!

Thursday, 1 April 1993
My amazing Perth sister, Geraldine! Snip, snip, stitch, stitch and I have a new wardrobe of seven pairs of trousers and one skirt as well as high-quality matching T-shirts from one of her factory haunts. This activity of hers is in between working three nights of shift work at a local hospital, rearing her three treasures of 4, 5 and 6, entertaining me and competently running her household, husband and dog. This 40-something sister of mine is the only one of my sisters to have produced any children. Because of that, her three are the closest to any blood children of mine. Therefore, precious and poignant.

Sunday, 11 April 1993
A family Easter. My Tasmanian sister and her husband are here too. I took a roll of cellophane to my mother's to roll off some for my Perth and for my Tasmanian sisters. This particular type of cellophane can be heat-sealed with a warm iron. It is thus useful to both of the above sisters who are great makers of interesting things that might need to be wrapped. We all seem to have a gene for 'I-want-some-too. I-think-I-need-it.' Mum likes to be in on the action too. She was watching me roll the cellophane from the large roll. Because I knew she wanted some and because her very indirect way of making requests annoys me, I decided to string her along a bit. The conversation went as follows:

> MUM: You're really good at rolling that up, Mary.
> ME: Mmmm.
> MUM: What do you use it for, Mary?
> ME: Wrapping, Mum.
> MUM: You're doing a good job, Mary.
> ME: Mmmmmm.
> MUM: Mary, who's that for?

ME: X, Mum. (The Perth sister.)
MUM: Are you doing some for Y? (The Tasmanian sister.)
ME: Yes.
MUM: You're very good at rolling it.
ME: Mmmmmm.
MUM: Mary. Do you think I could have just a little bit?

And so she did.

Tuesday, 27 April 1993
I don't want to go back to work. I don't want to work. Colander head is still in the ascendancy. When I hear others discussing matters academic it all floats right over the top of my head. I am at home with plenty of work to do. I have no motivation. I just want to sleep. I am also heavily into work-avoidance strategies. Quinces are in season, so I have spent hours at my stove making batches of quince paste. I make some, tell people about it, induce them to try it, give it all away and then have to make more.

I took some to Peter at the French stall at Vic Market. He asked me if I'd make some so he could sell it. 'No.' I said, 'I'm not a seller. I prefer to give things away.' So I couldn't find alternative employment in any kind of selling game. Then again I don't really want alternative or any employment. I just don't want to work. Will this change before the dreaded date in July when I go back to uni? This has probably been the longest period in my life when I have been left to my own resources. I'm not depressed about any of the above. It's as if it doesn't relate to me at all. I'm never bored when left to my own devices.

Saturday, 8 May 1993
Tomorrow I'll be 52. I've decided that I'm dying. Not just think or have any evidence for it. My father died when he was 52 years and 232 days old. He died unexpectedly. I'm the eldest child. When I reach 52 years and 232 days old I'll have a party on the next day (29th December). I'll know which side of the family my genes come from. I know it's quite an irrational fear but it's caused me to sort of freeze and not want to do anything. I'm not afraid

of dying. I just don't want it to happen yet. I've got too much to do and I don't even have a cemetery plot. During the week I woke up in the middle of the night — as usual — with the radio on — as usual. I think there was a radio play being broadcast — perhaps it was a dream. Anyway, the bit I heard included a segment where people were standing, commenting around the open coffin of a woman. I have no idea what it was all about. I must have gone back to sleep.

Sunday, 15 May 1993
I've just been monitoring my erratic behaviour. I'm supposed to be writing two learned? articles. At least I managed to get the computer turned on. That was at 9 a.m. It's now 2 p.m. Having turned on the computer I decided that answering letters was more urgent — some letters that I've had since January. I then discovered that I had separated the cards and letters from their envelopes and addresses. Hunt for these. In the process of going through four high piles of paper on my living-room table I become sidetracked. Ah, that's where that receipt went to. Where did I put the others? Off to another room to check another pile of paper. Then I wonder if those jumpers are dry yet? No, so I pull out a few weeds on the way inside from the washing line. I then have to wash my grubby hands. There are a few dishes to do. Perhaps I'll have a cup of tea. That will make me feel better. What was it I was doing? Oh yes — letters. It would be a good idea if I put all the addresses on the scrapbook on my computer. Then I wouldn't need all these bits of paper. That done but still no writing. I decide to clean out my handbag. If I'm having a clean out of bits of paper then why not do the handbag as well. Good idea. I end up with a plastic bag of rubbish and discover that I've lost (mislaid) the winning TAB ticket from yesterday — worth $30. Can't lose that. Tip out all the rubbish and go through it piece by piece. Not there. The said ticket was nestling in another pile of papers that were not to be thrown out. Three letters finally get written. I should put some photographs in some of the letters. Where are they? Another distraction while I find them. I should ring Mum. Do so, and she's busy. Says she'll ring back.

... Mum rings. Talk for ten minutes. I think I'd better make some soup and my neck needs a rest too. Do some neck exercises. Notice the uncompleted crossword on the kitchen table. If I'm throwing out paper I should throw out that newspaper too. I'll just see if I can solve a few more clues. How's the soup going? Time to eat some lunch. Perhaps I can watch channel two's Sunday program while I'm having the soup. I'll just check the jumpers again. The sky is becoming dark and overcast. Jumpers in, but still a bit damp. Don't want them to go out of shape. How can I hang them? A long piece of dowelling will do (9 feet long). Where can I place that? It will fit in the study from the top of the filing cabinet to the back of my chair. Knock over the chair. Start again. Mission successful. Soup and time for a rest.

Tuesday, 18 May 1993
I still have not remembered any dreams. I like the concept that dreams are the dustbin of the mind. Perhaps I don't want to remember any of mine. Perhaps I want to package them in plastic bags and throw them out each day when I dispose of my other rubbish.

Friday, 28 May 1993
I'm supposed to go to get a breast cancer X-ray, a-just-in-case one. I mentioned it to Mum one day. Her response, 'There's no history of breast cancer in our family Mary.' While she has a high regard for doctors — I think she places them above the angels in her scheme of things — she has a healthy scepticism about ailments. I have a degree of her cynicism too. So — perhaps I will. Perhaps I won't.

Monday, 31 May 1993
Almost winter. I've been thinking that maybe I'm just a malingerer. Maybe I need a proverbial boot-in-the-bum in the head. Then I remind myself that I've not been a malingerer before. I've always been a doer. I had expected that this menopausal transition would be a breeze. No worries and all that. But it hasn't. It's been horrid. I should have been more sympathetic in the past to women of this

age. Some of my older friends just shrug and say, 'Oh, I had no problems. Just the occasional hot flush.' An erstwhile colleague reminded me that my life has been full-on since I was 3 years old. Always another baby sibling to look after. Always a meal to cook for the others. But I always enjoyed those tasks. My mother loved school holidays because it meant that the children would be home with her.

I can remember my mother, seemingly always pregnant, struggling up the hill each Friday to the newsagent to buy me the next edition of *The Girl's Crystal* comic, the latest Billabong book or one of the Dimsie series. This latter series was set in snooty public English girls' schools, but I loved them nevertheless. I devoured books, good, bad and indifferent, though some of the Grimm's fairy tales and other stories of that ilk I still remember, and sometimes read again with great affection. My favourite is the one about the sister whose seven brothers were turned into swans. She was required to release them by spinning flax and making it into shirts for them. It was, as I remember, a torturous process during which blood dripped constantly from her fingers, she was overcome with fatigue but eventually overcame the curse and the pain. There has to be a message there somewhere.

Friday, 11 June 1993
A black thunder mood but no spark as there's no energy. I've been cooking and heard Jocelynne Scutt talking on the radio about her new book about women ageing. All these positive images of septuagenarians climbing mountains, chairing international conferences, being movers and shakers and only having the slightest difficulty when their bones creak and complain as they try to squat over oriental toilets. Fucking hell! I don't want to do any of that. I just want to be left alone. My other reading keeps saying how wonderful it is — to get old.

Sunday, 13 June 1993
I'm still thinking about what I'm passionate about or what really bugs me or would cause me deep grief. Nothing really. I don't get

fazed easily. I've lived with cannibals, seen lots of life and death — the latter is our only certainty, don't care much for money or prestige. Religion doesn't have a grip on me, New Age or otherwise, though I'm glad to have been brought up in a Christian tradition. The only saint I've ever had much time for is crazy Francis of Assisi. He didn't ever lose his sense of wonder. I heard Caroline Jones interviewing callers about an Ahaa they thought they'd experienced. Responses full of light coming in windows, dazzling smiles from significant others, near-death experiences while falling down crevasses etc., etc. When I was in New Guinea as an impressionable 20-something-year-old, I spent half my time meditating and being religious. Been there done that. A Mozart symphony, Cecilia Bartoli singing, a Beethoven concerto or a leaf in bud can really spin me out. What's a life worth?

Monday, 14 June 1993
A period. Imagine that. After none for about a year. I still had a sanitary pad in a drawer. It had occurred to me that I might frame the unused pad as a memory of things past. Anyway it explains my recent black thunder moods, the slowing down of the hot flushes and the black rings under my eyes. I wonder if it's my last egg to be dispersed into the universe. As David Suzuki says, everyone's molecules are all mixed up with everyone else's, from Moses to Mozart to me and my old eggs. Journey well, egg.

I began menstruating when I was about 11. I was ill prepared. My mother gave me a piece of elastic, two safety pins and a folded piece of white cloth. I didn't really know what it was all about. It wasn't until I was about 14 that I knew how sex really worked — just as a physical plumbing principle.

Migraines began at the time I started menstruating. I had been visiting a relation with my aunt. The relation served caraway-seed cake. I had a migraine and later threw up. I'm sure there was no causality but I haven't eaten caraway seed again to this day.

Thursday, 30 June 1993
Home again! Home again! Jiggety jig!

What have I been doing? I have been in Queensland. My primary purpose was to give a paper at a conference and to do some educational visiting. What else? I stayed at the Brisbane home of a past boarder here. He's now chief geologist at a gold mine. I visited the mine, met up with people I hadn't seen for years (some for twenty-five years), went on train journeys through the Glasshouse Mountains and boiled in the Queensland winter while the locals were clad in winter garb. Also did heaps of walking and reading. In fact I think I managed to turn some kind of mental corner. After I had read about ten books in three days — mostly, but not all, thrillers, I had to ask myself if a diet of cheap literary pulp was to sustain me for the rest of my days. No! No! No. There are other things in life. Tomorrow I go back to work.

Saturday, 10 July 1993
I have had a reprieve. I visited Mum as it was the anniversary of my father's death. We talked about him. I had thought his cause of death was a heart attack. (I was in New Guinea when he died.) No, said Mum. He had the flu. Because he was taking cortisone for his sarcoidosis, his resistance was lowered. He'd always had high blood pressure, took tablets (Veganin) as if they were Smarties all his life. The cause of death was listed as hypertension and pulmonary oedema. Later (ten years later), it was possible for her to get a war widow's pension because of the sarcoidosis and some rearrangement, by Legacy, of the causes of death. The Porters (my father and his sister) lived on tablets, said mother. I'm not like that. I don't have a history of hypertension. I have stopped counting the days to 29 December. I'll still have the party.

Mum had to go to the doctor as she has the flu. The doctor commented on Dad's relatively young age of death — he was 52. She was left with eleven children still at home. The doctor said it must have been difficult for her. She said 'Oh I never thought of it like that.' I genuinely believe that that's how it was, and still is, for her. It's just a matter of getting on with life. She really is an amazing woman. We've not really appreciated that in her.

Wednesday, 14 July 1993

Not as tired. Have more energy. I've been musing as I move objects around the home. A heavy-hand-spun woven woollen Welsh blanket, embroidery from India and Pakistan, linen and lace from China, artifacts from Korea and Japan. Nothing matches anything else. I must have been furnishing imaginary rooms/events in my mind. The blue blanket for a child's room, the embroidery for exotic dresses for grand occasions, the linen and serviettes for long and lavish meals, the boxes of brass handles and door furniture to decorate doors I could fling open with panache to welcome guests, all the culinary appurtenances jamming up my kitchen to enable me to transform raw produce into jewelled jars. However, I have also realised that these rooms can be furnished in my mind, and changed around, with great ease. Is there a fine line between living in cloud-cuckoo-land and having a healthy imagination?

Friday, 30 July 1993

Some reflections about the last year. I'm not sure if all my dismal episodes were exactly menopausal. I think I needed a break from work after three very, very hard years — I'm inured to hard years, but not to very, very hard ones. I'm not sure if I could have endured more of the same. How much of it was the need for a mental holiday/change of scenery, I don't know. Perhaps I was depressed. Certainly the symptoms — no, not a good descriptor, the indicators of ageing are with me. I think I can cope with them now. I guess we start ageing from birth but there are some express stations along the way. This period has been that. I'd still like to retire but I'm resigned to not being able to. I feel better about myself.

Saturday, 31 July 1993

Today I've been thinking about why people have children. I know several 30-something friends who would love to have a child but have not yet had the chance. (Our parents had no other option.) Do we consider it to be our biological destiny? To form a dynasty? To perpetuate ourselves? Do people want to see their mirror images? To cement a relationship? (Weak glue that.) Is it security against old age? Why do people assume that one takes a conscious decision to be childless. I think it should be looked at from the other perspective. It should be a conscious and considered decision to have, not to not have, them. I like children — how could I not? Streams of generations flow through my life continuously. How fortunate to be at such a confluence of times and cultures.

Thursday, 5 August 1993
. . . as for my teaching, I've decided that the best I can do is to teach people to think. There is no guarantee my students will get jobs. So, after all that, I had my students fill in an identity grid. They did this and I did one too, to enable them to see a contrast. Later, I chatted to the sociologists and the psychs in search of illumination about the concept of identity. I scoured the library for stuff on identity. Not much. I ended up with Erikson's model [identifying various life stages]. I've included my responses [to some of Carmel's questions]. They came straight off the top of my head. Later I realised that they could be related to what Erikson says. Here are the respones I made:
- *Where do I think I am now, relative to 12 months ago?* I'd still like to retire, but I can wear being at work.
- *Do I have any sense of transition?* I have been thinking about these questions and maybe my conclusion to the journal will answer some of them. Observing myself in this menopausal life process has been an interesting, if sometimes negative, learning experience. I am glad to have done it.

Today I had a long, rambly letter from the friend I met in Queensland recently. I hadn't seen her for twenty-five years. She reminded me that I'd told her about my parking-spot philosophy and about how she has begun to subscribe to it. I'd forgotten all about it. It's just this. I believe that whenever I need a place to park it will be exactly outside where I am going — 99.9% of the time it is. That's the philosophy I apply to my life. And it usually works.

Saturday, 7 August 1993
I have just returned from a wonderful wind-in-the-face-on-the-way, wind-on-my-wing-on-the-way-home bike ride. I was thinking about age during my small voyage. I thought about being old, dignified and graceful. No, that is not me. I treasure my eccentricity, so, no grace and dignity for me. I like me the way I am.

This has been the story of the beginning of one woman's journey (2-hour ticket, zone one) into old age — not a euphonious phrase, but a reality. I am unaware of all the sub-agendas in this encapsulated splinter of my life. (Like a relic of the true cross!) I am also unaware of all the levels at which I operate. Future reflection may help me to sort these out. However, it has been illuminating for me to write this journal.

7
PRIVATE PARTS IN PUBLIC PLACES

Nicole Davis, Carmel Seibold and Lyn Richards

> Hot flushes? . . . Quite frankly when I'm at work, I can't be bothered. I just loosen the front of my shirt and let the steam out . . . I often wonder what the other people in the meeting must think, because I'm going from one extreme to the other. But they don't last for more than a few minutes with me anyway, so they are no real problem . . . Quite frankly if you're busy and working, you've got your mind on other things; that may lessen it for you because you're so interested in other things you really haven't got the time to worry about what's happening with yourself . . . From talking to my mother and friends, I think if I was doing nothing at home — I'm not saying housewives do nothing, I'm being very, very careful here — but if I had less to do, I think probably you would think about it more, it might assume a greater importance. (Full-time, professional midlife woman.)

Sue, on the other hand, classed her hot flushes as not serious only because they occurred after she had left work:

> And I did have this advantage, yes, last year's bout as well as this year's bout, that I wasn't working. And I mean, that probably, that certainly would have reduced my stress levels a certain amount. And I wasn't sitting there in a room full of men in dark suits who wouldn't dream of taking their jackets off!

As another midlife women commented: 'If you're home, you can put up your feet. But if you're outside [at] work, you've got to put on this act all the time, and sometimes you can't put it on.'

MIDLIFE HAPPENS SOMEWHERE!

The previous chapters have shown that women are active agents in constructing their understanding of menopause, in the context of societal images. We focused first on the wider backdrop of social images, then on women's individual experiences. This chapter is about the contexts between. Social expectations and personal decisions take place in a more particular context, and a woman's placement will always affect her experience and her understanding of menopause. The processes of knowledge construction are always mediated not only by social images and individual agency but also by the woman's own place and social context. Women are always *somewhere*.

For any woman, her experience of midlife will depend on where she is, in many senses. Where is she physically — in an urban or rural place? Where is she socially, in an unequal society, and how does she see herself, her resources and opportunities? Where is she in a multicultural society, where ethnic origin may determine health knowledge, interpretation of body, and life chances? Where is she in a social network, of family, colleagues and friends?

In this chapter we address some of these questions by asking another: where is she in the two worlds of home and paid work, (still seen by most women as the private and public worlds)? Paid work proved a powerful theme. One of the clearest unexpected messages to emerge from our data was that whether or not a woman was or had been in paid work was always relevant to her story of midlife. Many women spoke as though their experience was above all determined by employment, its conditions and its contributions, positive and negative, to their lives. We had not asked directly about work at the start of the project, but in the preliminary analysis of the qualitative data it turned up more often than discussions of any other context except family. Work colleagues and their contributions, positive and negative, often took up more space than discussions of the contributions of partners. This was partly, we came to realise, because the context of women's work lives, whether at home or in the workplace, reflect and affect all other dimensions of their social contexts — location, networks, culture and class, resources and constraints.

MIDLIFE IN THE NINETIES

For all women now the personal experiences of midlife and menopause occur in public places. Whether or not they 'stay home', women are out of the home for much of their daily lives. However their lives in the workforce are more visible and less flexible than their home lives: women in the workplace are likely to find it harder to avoid going public, to dodge bad days, to reject as irrelevant to them the images of youth and vitality associated with success. The cohort of women now experiencing menopause has a higher rate of workforce participation and career commitment than any before,[1] and is most vulnerable to images of womanhood that combine, in complex ideologies, the twin ideals of nurturing motherhood on the one hand, youth, attractiveness, independence and sexuality on the other. At no other time in history has women's participation in paid work been a normal part of their life cycle.

For the cohort of women approaching and experiencing midlife in the 1990s, these contexts are dramatically different from those of their mothers. Midlife women, unlike previous generations of women are likely either to be experiencing menopause in the public arena of paid work or to be very aware of others doing so. They are likely to feel sharply the incompatibility of the dual duties of home and paid work: typically they entered full-time work only after having children, and with considerable social disapproval. Sue's story is typical of women entering the workforce in the seventies.

> I had started in 1979 at the stage when I was very much a part-time casual researcher working the hours which fitted in with the kids at school. I couldn't go back to work until they were both at school and

I then worked . . . nine to three on the days that I could [arrange these hours] . . . Well it was almost impossible then, I am talking about 1975! Nobody was employed on those terms, I was just lucky . . . But obviously that held me back in my career, but I wasn't concerned because my family was a priority and I was still of the old school. But also had a mother saying to me you really shouldn't be doing this.

In Western societies, this was a cohort for whom the escape from 'private' to 'public' sphere was fought and politicised. The relevance of paid work to women's experiences of midlife has hardly been explored in the literature. Kaufert (1982) argued that a woman's socio-economic status influences her experience of menopause because her status influences her work choices and hence her experiences. Traditionally consigned to the private sphere, women in the 1990s now combine family and work roles in increasingly complex ways. So they experience their major biological and social transitions in both 'worlds' and both will contribute to that experience. Unlike many other transitions, menopause is intensely private, involving physical change and belonging to the aspect of women's lives most associated with the private world of family — reproduction. Unlike other transitions, it can be kept secret, kept out of her experience of the world 'outside'. However this is far more difficult when she is daily in the spaces and social structures of the world of work. What are the contributions of family and work experiences to women's interpretation of their midlives?

This chapter starts with the responses from the survey to the question: do you think the midlife years will be easier or harder for women who do paid work? It then draws on five case studies, of women in different settings, to explore their unique stories in the shared contexts of spatial, social, and cultural location.

How does work work for women in midlife?

When we designed the survey, along with asking women whether they thought menopause would be easier or harder if in paid work, we also asked women how important their work was to them. A high proportion (70%) saw work as important to them. We were startled by the widespread conviction of work's relevance, and by the two faces work presented in the answers. Even though the majority of women reported that work was important to them, many did not feel that the midlife years would be made easier by work. Only 38% thought midlife would be easier if working. The midlife women's perception of its impact split between 'easier' and 'harder'. One of the reasons women felt paid work would make one's midlife either easier or a bit easier was because work could offer a welcome distraction from changes occurring in their bodies and their lives. Some typical comments from the survey were:

> As I believe in keeping busy, it seems to help if you don't have too much time to think about it.
>
> While working it keeps your mind off midlife.
>
> Some days if I hadn't had a job I could [have] shot myself. That is the truth — I felt so low some days.
>
> If you are busy you won't worry about midlife as much, also financially it makes it easier.

Work was also seen as offering rewards relating to women's sense of self-esteem, personal satisfaction and companionship:

> Because you [are] not so isolated as you might be at home.
>
> It takes your mind away from the home, and you are meeting people.
>
> Focus other than self. Reward, esteem, sense of self reinforced by professional identity.
>
> Independence/companionship/sense of worth.
>
> Personal satisfaction of doing a job well and supporting yourself during a self-doubting unsure period of time.
>
> Midlife years for women who are working are much easier because they feel useful and needed.

Many women from the survey commented on the financial rewards that work provided in midlife:

> You should have money for some little extras in life for yourself and children and partner.

So you don't have to worry [about] how you are going to cope financially, as much as if you were not working.

Other women were working out of sheer economic necessity, and not just to supplement the family income: 'If I don't work I don't eat.'

Some women commented that because their children were older and not dependent on them, working at midlife was easier than it had been previously: 'Children old enough to help around the home, to look after themselves after school etc.' Women who thought that work made midlife harder related their comments to tiredness and trying to balance family and work. Twenty-seven per cent of all the surveyed women thought that paid work would make the midlife years a bit harder and 7% believed it would make them much harder. The midlife women commented as follows:

> Because I'm up at 5 a.m., leave 6 a.m., home 6.30 p.m., then do housework — my biggest problem [is] tiredness. But then again without the money — many other problems would arise.

> Work and housework equals always tired.

> As we get older I think we seem to need more rest. When we are younger we seem to get by on less sleep, relaxation etc.

> Having to hold down a job to support family while feeling unwell or unhappy due to menopause. Also more pressure to keep that job.

The dual role of all women but particularly midlife women was referred to in the survey in relation to making work at midlife harder:

> People slow down but still have to go to work and run a home.

> Well a woman works hard whether it is outside the home or if it is in the home.

> More physically demanding [midlife and coping with home duties] for me as a manual worker.

Women also reported the pressure to perform relative to younger colleagues, along with keeping a job when ageing, as factors that make working at midlife harder. Performance was measured by some of the women surveyed in comparison with the young, fit and responsibility free:

> We live in a youth-oriented society where age is considered a handicap, not an asset.
>
> Who wants to employ someone close to retirement?
>
> We are being replaced by younger, more educated people all the time.

The women responding to the survey suggested that no allowances are made for menopausal women and that there was no time to adjust to the changes they were experiencing: 'Because the side-effects of midlife and having to work each day puts added pressure on the woman and does not allow time to rest, adjust or seek help.'

Another woman spoke not only of the changes happening to her body which impacted on her working life, but also of changes in her personal life: 'A marriage separation which is placing stress on my body. Had to have a colposcopy [due to an] abnormal smear test. [It] worries me that my body will react negatively to all this stress.'

Some of the survey respondents made the point that liking one's job, being content in one's personal life, having a symptom-free menopause and a positive outlook had a bearing on whether work would be easier or harder for midlife women:

> All depending on how contented you are with life and depending on whether you are happy with your work paid or unpaid.
>
> Depends on type of menopause i.e. heavy bleeding and pain etc.
>
> I believe that mental attitude plays a huge role in the physical well-being and that some people [are preconditioned] to expect a hard time.

The following sections will explore a number of the themes identified in the survey data through the stories of five midlife women. Areas not addressed in the survey responses, namely support from families and work colleagues, will also be examined.

THE WOMEN'S STORIES

Lena is married, her husband of two years is a professional and she is aged in her early forties. She has three adult children from her previous marriage all of whom have moved out of home. She is an intelligent, career-oriented woman who works at a senior management level for a large computer company. She sees herself as pre-menopausal. Her house suggests that she lives a very comfortable upper-middle-class life. Lena points out that her family life is different from many women she knows as she has recently married:

> I think it's probably different for us. We've only been married two and a half years. So, he's not the father of the children. It's not an issue for us, and it's not an issue anyway. Basically I think he's been a wonderful man to soldier through somebody else's teenagers . . . We probably go out on our own if we can, because we enjoy each other's company. I don't think it's different for my husband. I have one or two good friends and we see them occasionally. But, basically, we go out on our own. I think the only concern I have is my husband is too dependent on me. He doesn't do his own thing.

Sue's story, by contrast, is one of those we have termed as showing transition work. She is disengaging from her professional career, has changed jobs and is currently not working. At the time of the interview she was 48, living with her professional husband in an elegant house that seems designed for a couple. Her children have left home.

Mavis is married and her husband is self-employed as a handy man. She is aged in her late forties and has two adult children who have left home. Mavis lives in an inner working-class suburb and the data suggest she has a comfortable life and a strong relationship with her husband. She has recently retired from working in a gas-fitting factory and was, at the time of interview, experiencing some symptoms that could be termed menopausal. Mavis feels that leaving work has allowed her to regain her health:

> I had an awful lot of back problems again. I suffered with all those problems, headache, back problems until about one and a half years ago. Gradually being home for over two years [it] has taken me that long to get rid of all the tension in [my] life. I don't get headaches, although I have high blood pressure, but that's probably heritage, because my mother had high blood pressure, and my sisters have high blood pressure.

Sonia is married to a younger man who works as a nurse. She is aged in her early forties, has two children aged 8 and 10, and works part-time as an administrative assistant. The family income is under $50 000 and she lives in a traditionally working-class area that has recently become sought after by educated couples with an interest in older homes. She says she is experiencing menopause. She reported there was a point in her marriage where she contemplated separation, but later in the interview she said she questioned its value after visiting the Department of Social Security. This economic bind is common for many women who have young children and are in relationships which they see as less than satisfactory:

> My marriage is a fairly difficult one. It always has been. There has been a lot of arguments which came to a head at Easter this year. A lot of it is to do with my husband's background. Low self-esteem came from . . . his father [who] was an alcoholic and he grew up with verbal abuse and that has carried over to our family somewhat. What happened at Easter this year made me . . . Well I actually did go to Social Security to find out how I would stand if we did separate. I have often thought over the last years really, we could be better friends if we didn't live together. But I think I have come to the realisation this year that it is a marriage that shouldn't fail but might. I think we are actually on better terms now than we have been for a while . . . As far as our sex life is concerned, well that's dropped off a lot in the last few years. I have a mental interest in sex but not particularly physical.

While Sonia's situation may appear distinctive (in regard to the age of her children and her menopausal status), changing demographics will see an increasing number of women married with young children and experiencing midlife and menopause.

Karla (one of the women introduced in chapter 4) is aged 46 and divorced. She has two children aged 16 and 14 and works full-time combining her work as an independent nurse practitioner with agency work. She sees herself as menopausal. Karla, like Sonia, is still very enmeshed in caring for dependent children. Although her children are in their teens she talks about balancing her private and public lives:

> It's hard to try and be there for the children, there for the job and still

have some life of your own. I think sometimes *my* [private] life is on hold. It's very hard to find the energy to put into a relationship on top of kids and work.

WHAT DOES WORK DO FOR MIDLIFE?
THE PRESSURE TO PERFORM — IMAGES AND ENERGY

The impact work has on women's midlife experiences will depend on the type of work. Physical work will put a greater strain on the body but having to perform in public in a professional capacity can also make balancing work and menopause very difficult. Pressure means different things to women in different work situations.

Each of these five women talked of work as pressure, and felt midlife and menopause was both harder and easier for women in paid work. However their reasons for it being harder were different because the pressure was different according to where they were in work and the workplace.

Lena, as a senior manager, feels she is constantly being evaluated in terms of her work performance. Menopause, she thought, was 'harder to handle' in the workplace because of the labelling by colleagues:

> I think people make judgments about middle-aged emotional women. I'm damn sure they do. You can cry at 21 and it's okay. If you cry at 45 or 50 . . . 'we all know why she's crying'.

Potential pressure on her, as a midlife woman, came, she said, from younger men and women's inability to cope with midlife women. The environment of the high-tech industry in which she worked may have contributed to her perceptions:

> I think it's a great problem for women who work for younger women [and men]. And, I've seen it twice in my career. I think they feel threatened, because they . . . I think they find it difficult, which consequently would come back on yourself. I think you are very much being judged . . . not exactly embarrassment to them, but they don't know how to cope.

Sue, who moved to an equal employment opportunity (EEO)

position in her forties, also found the pressure to perform exhausting:

> You actually can't stay in EEO for very long there is a real burn-out factor, it is life in a fish-bowl. It's walking around an organisation and having smart-alec men all the time asking you questions like, 'You still doing that silly job?' Snide remarks all the time to me at meetings. And generally the pressures of being where there is trouble all the time and not being able to rectify it . . . I had to constantly push myself to the fore for action, bold and noisy, and make sure there was a fortnightly column in the organisation newsletter and put up with all the hate mail that emanated as a result of what I wrote, and remain jovial and happily get up and talk to 200 people at a meeting and constantly display myself which isn't my natural inclination . . . So after 18 months I thought I think I have had enough.

Even though Sue works in the EEO area she still battles discrimination on a personal level. After leaving she ruefully expects the image of midlife to hinder her re-employment:

> There is a slightly worrying tone to the notion . . . of turning 50. Of course I am not actually in a stable job situation. I mean I am in a situation where next year I may well be applying for jobs and I am conscious that 50 on a CV doesn't look as good as 49 so I have got another unrealistic anxiety associated with that, but I don't have any sort of generalised anxiety about the number yet.

Karla captures the sheer exhaustion experienced by many midlife women who also feel vulnerable as a result of their age and their menopausal status:

> I love my work but I feel constantly under pressure to perform. What if I get sick? What if it falls on top of me? When I first realised I was menopausal I kept it to myself. I thought people would label me and I was trying to establish myself — I needed to be seen as energetic and coping.

Mavis, who with a less-visible profile on the factory floor had her performance evaluated by how much stock she produced, was under pressure of a different kind. She had worked in a factory for most of her thirties and early forties, and described a conflict between her body's needs and those of the workplace:

I had very demanding work in my early thirties, and I carried that job through for ten years without much problem healthwise. But, I noticed at 38 I was . . . I just felt that I couldn't settle into . . . I felt if I had to work harder than I did it depressed me . . . I felt that my body was screaming out 'I don't want this anymore.'

She chose to listen to her body and retire in her mid-forties. Although she acknowledged the physical strain work placed on her in midlife, in retrospect she recognises the positive benefits of remaining physically active: 'I suppose I slowed down a bit . . . once you start sitting down, I think your body takes on a different approach about everything.'

TIME AND TIREDNESS

Neither Lena nor Mavis had anything to say about the impact of menopausal symptoms on their working lives, but rather spoke in terms of a body ageing physically and visually. However Sonia and Karla did note the effect of such symptons. Both talked about the difficulty of managing work and family with dependent children. Sonia, for example, felt that coping with menopausal symptoms was much harder for working women:

> It was complicated in my case having young children at the crèche. It was certainly difficult. A lot of depression, tension, extreme PMT. . . One of the symptoms I had was extreme insomnia. Particularly that first year. And you come to work on two hours sleep. Come in to work a full day and then deal with kids at night. That was the worst I think.

Karla saw work as both her salvation and a great stress. The stress related to performing adequately in order to provide an income. She reflects the vulnerability of many single midlife women. Her single status makes her reliant on a regular income to support herself and her children: 'If there's one word to describe my life it's exhaustion, sheer bloody exhaustion. But I know I have to keep running round that wheel. No one else is going to spell me.'

Managing symptoms

The need to manage one's body in the workplace becomes of paramount importance to most women who experience physical changes that are visible. Their discussions of managing symptoms are almost entirely about flooding or hot flushes. And these discussions usually involve the decision to commence HRT or to continue taking it. Karla was referring to experiences leading up to her decision to take HRT when she recounted an experience of flooding at work (quoted in chapter 4, p. 56). She remembers this as acutely embarrassing despite the fact she was addressing health workers: 'You feel you no longer have control over your body.'

Another reason Karla gave for choosing to take HRT was to deal with tiredness:

> I was so tired all the time what with waking up at night. Not that I had the dreadful hot flushes that some women complain about but I did feel anxious and just drained of energy. HRT did help. It helped me cope with work, kids, the whole catastrophe.

It is possible that Karla would have chosen to take HRT whatever her circumstances, however, the theme of coping at work and coping with the dual demands of work and family was very evident in her decision.

Sonia takes hormone tablets and while she doesn't relate her decision to coping at work, she does comment that it is to alleviate her symptoms, which had made managing work and family extremely difficult:

> I take Ogen tablets which are oestrogen That is a whole tablet from day five to day twenty-five of the cycle. I take half a progesterone tablet. That is Provera, from day fifteen to day twenty-five. I have an oestrogen implant. That is a 50 milligram implant every five months. Originally it was six months but I found that the last few weeks I was getting the symptoms back again so I cut it back to five months. That has made enormous differences.

Sonia feels good about taking hormones, especially in relation to the improvement in her quality of life:

I know he is right [her doctor]. I mean no matter what his critics say — he has a lot of critics. He might be wrong on plenty of other things but he is right on this one [taking hormones].

WORK AS NETWORK

Work did not necessarily provide all women with an intimate, sharing place. Rather the emphasis across much of our data is on ways of not revealing weakness at work, and this is true of women in all positions. One medical employee went to a clinic at another hospital because she didn't want anyone at her hospital to know she was menopausal. You can talk about affairs and family dramas, but not things that might make you seem less competent. There was a sense that you need to make a public world and cling to your public image, especially for those women who were trying or had taken a while to reach a stable employment level.

But going to work, and being seen as competent at work, was critical in many women's self images. Even when they were ambivalent about the demands that work placed on the body, work was seen by a majority of women in the survey and by Lena, Sue, Mavis, Sonia and Karla as a source of social support. Social support was found in both friendship and less intimate contact such as a greeting on arrival:

> KARLA: Work does get you out of yourself. If you've had a blazing row with a teenage son going to work stops you brooding . . . did I say, did I do the right thing? You can compare notes with others with teenage kids.

Paradoxically work, while providing social support, can also mitigate against other forms of social contact. Time and energy considerations play a part. Sonia said:

> Oh well my social life is basically at work. With young children we don't go out very much anyway . . . but I guess a major factor in whether you enjoy your work is the people you know there . . . I have very few friends and that is probably why my husband and family mean a lot to me.

Lena's emphasis, rather than being on the constraints both

young children and work place on her, is on the need to conserve energy in the face of a demanding job:

> Social life . . . I have the sort of job where you are talking to people all day long and the phone drives me berserk, so if the phone rings [at home] I say it's not for me . . . I have one or two good friends and we see them occasionally. But basically we go out on our own.

For Lena, life centred around her work and her husband. However, given other professional women's accounts, it is likely that Lena, due to her seniority in the workplace, would draw support through networking with other professional women at work-affiliated functions.

The workplace, while providing the opportunity for friendship networks for some, can also provide other forms of support. For example, Karla's wide network of colleagues and health professionals provided support of a different type validating her as a competent person: 'I did not want support as a menopausal woman. I got support through their professional regard for me.'

However, women who are geographically isolated and travel long distances to their workplace can miss out on support at work and social contact outside of work. This was particularly so for women in rural or semi-rural areas, where resources of income and education did not protect against the 'tyranny of distance'. In the case of the Peninsula study referred to in the introduction, location and time were the critical factors in relation to establishing and maintaining a friendship network (Lewis 1996). One woman in the Peninsula study had commenced a new job at the time she started menopause. She considered that there had been no time to establish and develop the sorts of friendships in the workplace that would allow the kind of intimate sharing related to midlife health. In addition, although there were some women in the workplace, it was male-dominated. The job entailed working in three different locations approximately thirty minutes drive apart. This combined with the fact that she resided on a farm at some distance from any of these locations made involvement in either casual or more intimate sharing of menopausal symptoms and problems difficult. She revealed she had only one close friend whom she saw only occasionally. The rural nature of her residence ensured no casual neighbourhood contact over the back fence and the commuting distance to the three city workplaces limited any 'time out' for personal matters. Time in the context of location is significant when it is at a premium. In this woman's situation, travelling to work becomes time wasted, so location became the constraining factor that prevented her attending to her personal needs. Not only was she located in a geographically isolated area in terms of neighbourhood community, but also in relation to her workplaces.

Network maintenance can be made more difficult by both geographical distance and time. Mavis, for example, found this on retirement to a distant suburb, which often goes hand-in-hand with retirement from work. Distance interfered with contact from old friends: 'Of course it has changed, because we've made a move . . . I wish I could see more of my old friends but I suppose it has to be give and take, because of the distance.'

Sue's experience in leaving a workplace to which she had been very devoted startled her. But it also presented new opportunities. Sue's experience illustrates how support once found at the workplace often does not extend past one's working life even if the friendships had appeared more than casual:

> When I first went on leave and came back from overseas I still felt very much a part of the organisation and so when people rang me up and said, 'So and so is going off to have her baby, we're having a lunch', or 'So and so is leaving' — there were quite a lot of leavings because the organisation then offered redundancy packages . . . I went back to the office and listened to the chatter and the banter and so forth. I found myself each time more and more distanced from it and I saw myself sitting there feeling like an outsider, watching it and feeling 'Who would want to be a part of this?' So it was after a few months that I realised actually that there was no place for me back there.

Interestingly she found considerable pleasure in the casual contacts at her place of voluntary work, undertaken during her leave:

> It was a wonderfully freeing feeling to walk in there and be treated like a member of staff . . . although I was only there once a week I felt to some extent — in fact I was quite surprised [at] the extent to which I'd

wander in [in] the morning and head for the tearoom or the kitchen, tearoom is a rather glamorous word for those sorts of set-ups . . . and be greeted warmly by various people . . . and join in the chatter and eventually after a few weeks begin to discover that some of the gossip even meant something to me so I had a sort of de facto involvement in . . . a work group.

Family and work

For women for whom work consumes a lot of time and energy, family is supposed to be a haven of peace and support. But for those women with dependent children, family can be a burden and a cause of stress. For women who have support from partners and family it can be a positive place. For women whose parents were ageing or for women who assumed the role of maintaining the family links, midlife family caring and midlife work seem inextricably linked in their stories.

Karla, since her divorce, has placed great importance upon her family of origin to provide her with a sense of belonging and a place to seek intimacy. While her children were important they provided minimal support and were 'not much help after a hard day at work, more likely to add to my stress'. Her sister had taken the place of her partner as her close confidante: 'My family have been very supportive in an emotional sense, particularly my sister — she got me through, gets me through, the bad times.'

The others, all still married, named their husbands as their key support person but with somewhat different emphasis on the importance of this relationship. Mavis said: 'I have a very supportive husband, so, I can talk to him about anything, and I think that helps. I feel very secure there.'

Even though Sonia had experienced difficult times in her marriage, she still felt that her family and husband were central support anchors:

> I think that is a factor [seeing her husband as a friend]. It might be a fact of my own family background. You tend to choose a person that is not unlike your own parent. Yeah and I did have an active sex life with a number of people before I met my husband. There were two or

three after marriage. And I have always had more sex with other people. Not with strangers but on a short-term basis, much more exciting than with a long-term relationship. On the other hand, the long-term relationship is good for friendship, for children etc . . . From a sexual point of view, I'm not basically monogamous. But from a friendship point of view, I tend to be a bit of a loner.

Sonia indicates that her mother had been a major source of support until her death several years ago. The issue of family contact was complicated by her father's remarriage. She expressed her sense of dislocation occurring as a result of her mother's death, her estrangement from her father and her potential loss of links with the past. Since the breakdown of her extended family, Sonia emphasises the need for support from her husband as she doesn't have anyone else.

Sue's mother had died recently and the year of her illness had been a year of major disruption in Sue's work world. The two are strongly intertwined in her account. For some women, reaching the peak of their career coincides with parents reaching an age where they are fragile, often sick or dying:

> She died last year and [during] the last three years of her life she dominated every moment of mine . . . It was a dreadful year . . . I vacillated between full-time and thirty hours a week . . . I'd spent fifteen years in a government department in research . . . Certainly at 40 it was probably the stage [at] which I had got to the pinnacle of my work in that area. Work was pretty good and I think I was at that point [where] I had to go full-time, because there was no other way of carrying the responsibility I was carrying.

She sought and won a twelve-month secondment to another area which was less demanding and allowed her to cope with her dual roles:

> I had no intention of putting my research behind. I just wanted a break and . . . I had all sorts of notions of what could be achieved and I don't know whether I achieved any of them but one of the things I did discover was that actually you can't go back in life. After three months I rang my previous boss and said, 'Look I don't want to make things inconvenient for you running temporary fill-ins, I don't intend to come back.'

Family events again intervened, with a planned trip to England to see her father, long-divorced from her mother:

> So we planned the trip and my father then promptly died before I saw him ... and my mother then died in March and I really fell apart a bit, I found life terribly difficult, I was quite devastated for a while ... But ... it was also a new freedom, Dick's mother had died the year before and all of a sudden our kids had gone. One of them was starting to create enormous headaches for us ... and so basically I was feeling terribly traumatised and as my long service leave came up I'd also just started this Graduate Diploma ... as an attempt to try and just take myself right away from my work. I didn't like the difficulties with my mother, they were really the two factors in my life and I thought I'll just do a course, any course ... It was the worst year of my life, all of this came from the job. So May came, I was fascinated by the course, I was devastated by my mother's death, devastated by my daughter's problems and I thought I won't just make this my long service leave, I'm going to take a year's leave of absence, I can't give a stuff about this job.

Sue found distraction from work and family in an extension of work — study. Women who need to work for economic survival cannot take this option and like Karla, have to keep balancing family and work, with the concomitant potential for exhaustion and burn out.

CHOICE AND OPTIONS

For Sue, her social position allowed a choice about work, at least in economic terms. She was promoted, in a highly fluid workplace. 'It turned out to be horrible', and she stayed only eighteen months:

> I think I have done my, I was going to say done my dash with the public sector, bureaucracy — that is not true I was very disillusioned with the organisation, the organisation was going through hell, everyone was disillusioned, I was fortunate in that I had a way out. Most people just can't walk out of their job and say 'I'll take a year'. I was privileged in that I have got a husband who is quite capable of supporting me and quite willing to, so I thought I'll take twelve months, I'll travel, I'll see some friends, I'll go back to some music, I'll concentrate on my course and maybe I'll go back or maybe I won't.

She didn't. But while on leave she reflected on the lack of choice she had experienced and the new freedom of doing voluntary work. Midlife, and its changes, she sees as being easier if experienced out of the workforce:

> They're easier because I have got some time out and I am really, able to stand back, I mean I was sucked into a whole heap of what I can only describe as shit in the workforce. I was into status and I enjoyed my high salary and I enjoyed the prestige and being one of the women in a senior management position and I was so hooked in it that despite the fact that I didn't like it there was no way I could leave it, and having made the decision that these things don't matter a crumpet I feel a lot happier. So not being in the paid workforce is a wonderful freedom I have. I have had some wonderful choices about what to do with my time. I have been doing a lot of things that I want to do for no money!

One of the pleasures is in being able to choose her voluntary work:

> I didn't have to do anything — I chose to do something. When somebody said to me 'Do you want to run a course?' I said 'Sure' and they said 'What do you want to run a course in?' and I said, 'Yep sure okay.' 'There is one scheduled for next week do you want to do that one?' 'No I think I would rather do the one the week later' . . . and it was just wonderful to not feel under any obligation and just deliver of my best.

Obviously such choice is located in the social structure. For many women it seemed that work imposed a framework on their lives that could not be avoided or escaped. For other women this lack of framework meant poverty or deprivation both in and out of relationships. It is clear that Sue is in a select group of women who can afford and have support to take time out. Women who belong to the opposite end of the scale, who are in low-paying jobs or unemployed, do not have such choices. Karla, who works as a professional and has the capacity to earn enough money to adequately support herself and her children, sees herself as one of the lucky ones. When comparing Karla's and Mavis's situations — in terms of choice to work — it would appear that Mavis is not doing as well as Sue but is better off than Karla, in this regard. Much of the difference is based on expectations relating to desired lifestyles, for example, Mavis did not assume that her children would attend a university and require her support as Karla did. Karla, as a single mother, speaks of the pressure this imposes on her:

> I have no choice but to keep working and I'm one of the lucky ones. At least I can support myself and the kids — more or less. I have some status. Occasionally I envy the women on the supporting parent's benefit. They seem to be able to get to the gym! But then I play the Pollyanna game. Occasionally though I think it's not fair to have worked almost all your life and still be struggling to get by. We'd all like some 'time out'.

None of these women made a transition at midlife. But all of them were in some way shifted by it, and for all of them work was critical. Sue sees herself as changing in her values and her lifestyle, but not as doing the changing: 'I feel that I have been buffeted around a lot by external events rather than anything that has been internally driven or age-driven.' The changes are not solely to do with work, but work is involved in all of them, tangled with the demands of home and family.

> Actually I have moved into a phase of life where I appreciate solitude altogether . . . This was perhaps [due to] the frenetic way we lived our life and in between I rushed around to mum's and I felt that I was really achieving something because I was part of a busy social group and fulfilling all my obligations as a daughter, and mother and worker, and I suppose I was [affected by the] superwoman type thing.

Freedom from the public world

It has been clearly established in feminist writing that women never escape from the public world to a private haven. Family and work intertwine: the private world is invaded by the state and the economy, by patriarchy and violence; the family is a site of work and surveillance (Richards 1995). So we should not be surprised to find that work is relevant to women's private experiences of midlife. But its centrality did surprise us. Women's bodily changes are now in the public arena with the debate over medical treatments. And their accounts of the world of work and the need to escape from it indicate that having attained a place in the workforce, women at midlife often found that it was an uncomfortable place to be.

In this chapter we have described some processes of transition work: control of change, deliberate taking of time out from pressures to reassess self. In all our cases in which women spoke of taking control in this way, a part of the drama, and often the setting for it, was paid work. In all cases the two major issues were the visibility of private experiences in the workplace and the building pressure of multiple demands and inflexible timetables. And the only stories we have of women controlling the changes in their work lives were when they left. This is not, of course, to claim menopause causes women to leave paid work. But it hints at women's inability to find flexible workplace conditions and expectations to enhance their work lives, or even to control them, at times of personal and family stress.

The survey data, the case studies and Mary's story in chapter 6 clearly show that at midlife, as in earlier life stages, work has many meanings to women — just as it does to men (Harper & Richards 1978). However it could be argued that the needs of midlife women in the workforce are very different from those of younger women and of men. Their workforce careers and the associated pressures inextricably link with family caring whether of dependent children or parents. This is the cohort that won the battle for support of women when they entered the workforce: provision of adequate infant daycare is now considered a right, and maternity leave an obligation. But ironically at the age of double-burden caring, for both younger and older generations, there is no support in the workplace and the label of midlife menopausal woman is feared and the physical changes that provide evidence for it are dreaded. When pressures build up, the workplace provides no 'time out'. One clear conclusion can be drawn from both the survey and the qualitative data: for those in the paid workforce, the key to managing work and midlife relates to having flexibility in the workplace.

The experiences of this cohort of women will be the beginning of a knowledge base from which younger generations of women can learn. Their accounts contribute insights about the impact of work status and work conditions, and about the improvement of those conditions and the options available to deal with menopause, valuable information which can be used to understand the importance of the public context on the private experience.

Work is not the only public arena within which menopause and its experiences are potentially visible. The following chapters are concerned with another, the public health debate. As several previous chapters have shown, menopause is an increasingly high-profile public health issue: knowledge about it is public, and to get knowledge women have to go public. During the years of our project, menopause was increasingly being portrayed as a public health issue — a medical problem not an individual experience. Within one generation it was turned from a private experience contained within women's worlds of family to a public one.

We turn in the chapters that follow to the processes by which menopause is redefined as a medical and health policy problem surrounded by public controversy and delineated by medical discourse.

8
NATURAL AND UNNATURAL RISK — MIDLIFE AND WOMEN'S HEALTH

Claire Parsons and Val Seeger

SUSAN (35–39): Cervical cancer . . . I'm checked every year, and I . . . had a positive test about three years ago, . . . so I make sure I have a regular pap smear, I sort of feel as though I won't get breast cancer because my cousin, a close friend, a lady at work and someone else in the last month have all had their breasts removed. I think I've seen my fair share of one in ten or whatever it is around me, though I must admit I rushed out and had my mammogram two or three weeks ago . . . oh, it was just horrifying. Particularly as in two of the cases of cancer there were no lumps at all, they were picked up on routine mammograms, and it was an intraductal sort of cancer, that is, not a lump . . . and that really shocked me. I didn't know that. I had always associated breast cancer with lumps. If you can't feel any lumps you're fine — and that's just not true . . . I think a lot of women out there wouldn't know that.

THE RESEARCHERS

In 1994 our interest in the related concepts of women's health, health screening and risk had peaked. Here we were, Claire as a public health researcher with a multidisciplinary background in sociology, anthropology, nursing and medicine, Lyn as a sociologist, and Val with many years of nursing experience — all three facing or participating in the very subject under investigation.

Claire had been writing on the topic of 'risk and health' for the previous five years, while Lyn had experience in family research and had been working on a project to study the phenomenon of menopause. We decided to pool interests under the rubric 'women's health' and in 1993 were awarded an Australian Research Council grant.

Val launched herself daily into the morning's traffic, charting the maps to identify addresses, making friendships with strangers, accepting the hospitality of the women who had volunteered their time to be interviewed. Another social researcher, Maureen, entered the scene for a brief period to interview women in her 'neck of the woods'. We were seeking their stories and the women thrilled us with their narratives. These were the real life experiences of women forging their pathways through the chimera of an organised life — making sense out of the bits of living that we link up in our minds as a coherent (though in reality, fragmented) life story. We were privileged to be able to listen to the private lives of women anticipating or experiencing that misnomer we call 'midlife'.

THE WOMEN

We interviewed 167 women between the ages of 35 and 60 years, resident in three suburbs of Melbourne. The first was Kew with its upper-middle-class facade, the second Preston with its mix of middle and lower-class frontage, and the third Werribee with its predominantly working-class image. Of course, class as a sociological concept has done little to identify the thoughts, meanings and actions of women. We know women are not constrained by the usual indicators of class, such as education and income, whereby on the basis of 'good looks' a woman may be launched into the high life of a fashion model or may plunge into poverty through marital failure. Furthermore, irrespective of gender,

Australia has always sat uncomfortably within those historical continuities of the British class system.

In this study, the range of women's household incomes was reported as: less than $25 000 (23%), between $25 000 and $50 000 (35%), between $50 000 and $75 000 (23%), between $75 000 and $100 000 (10%), and 4% with over $100 000 per annum. Some did not identify their yearly household income. Of course, it is not clear from these figures if all the women had free access to this income, nor how many others were dependent on it. Using the Australian Bureau of Statistics classification of occupations, 24% of the women were professionals, 10% semi-professionals, 25% white-collar workers, 3.6% blue-collar workers, 1% students, and the rest (36.4%) carried on home duties. Well over half the women, despite their professional or white-collar worker status, lived in households with an annual income of less than $50 000.

Culturally, 131 were English-speaking in origin (Australian or other), of whom 101 related primarily to Anglo-Celtic culture and 24 to a mixed cultural background, while 33 were from non-English speaking backgrounds, of whom 18 identified most closely with a culture other than Anglo-Celtic (there were 3 non-responses).

These were women who gave of their time to disclose their losses and triumphs and personal perceptions as they responded to our questions about what the terms 'midlife' and 'risk' meant to them; they showed us how they made decisions about managing their health, their bodies and their minds. We sought to identify what type of knowledge these women had gained and the source, as well as how such information influenced their decision-making and where they were situated in the context of the competing discourses on women's midlife experience.

In this chapter, the concepts of midlife risks, health screening and disease prevention, and decision-making associated with perceptions of natural and unnatural risks, are illuminated through the narratives of these women; narratives that reflect their diversity of age, experience and values.

MIDLIFE RISKS

The women were asked what the term 'midlife' meant to them and about any risks they associated with midlife. The women responded to the first question in ways that emphasised the negative imagery and experiences associated with this life stage, using such descriptors as crisis, uncertainty, fear, getting older and recognition of one's own mortality. However, the occasional positive descriptor was also used, including being more confident, relaxed, children leaving the home and women being able to retrieve their own identities, or pursue their own interests.

Tamara is in her early forties and projects the images of negativity present in the media, declaring, 'I think midlife is something frightening if you don't know very much about it.' Mandy, who is in the same age range, says, midlife is 'scary. Somebody who is going off their head.' Eleanor is in her late forties and has witnessed friends undergoing difficulties associated with midlife changes. She responds to the question about what she thinks of when she thinks of the term 'midlife' by saying, 'Yes, quite neurotic type of problems. A lot of anxiety.' Perceptions of midlife often portrayed this life stage as bodies and minds starting to move down the slippery slide to chaos, bodies and minds out of control; although many felt that women could take some control over the pace of decline.

Camille, a woman in her early forties, responds to the term 'midlife' using common cultural representations, as she reports the threats or risks to the body and mind as somewhat controllable:

> First thought is, old age, wrinkles, hot flushes and turning 50. There are some things I do enjoy. I have more confidence at 43 than I did at 33 but with all the help you can get I don't think old age will be until I turn 60. I won't be old but I will be in old age. I'll be a senior citizen.

Responses offered variations on the theme of physical and mental deterioration, for while a number of the women mentioned their increased maturity and confidence at this life stage, they also reported concerns about physical and mental decline. It was not always clear which were attributable to physical changes and which to sociocultural changes, which has seen midlife become a time of maximum responsibility for others often coinciding with a peak in occupational performance and seniority. Life demands seem to be at a premium during the decade and a half when an individual is in her late thirties to early fifties, the time when menopause, as midlife physiological change, is often attributed with physical and mental decline in women:

> RUTH (35–39): Someone going through their midlife crisis, or midlife somewhere . . . around 40, or 40 to 50.
> HEATHER (50–54): Midlife, I don't know, I guess you think of grey hair . . . women that are becoming plump, oh I don't know, perhaps sometimes almost uninteresting people . . . a lot of the vitality that you have in your youth is . . . they're not as active, but probably that's a fallacy nowadays, I don't know.
> SACHA (50–54): Oh, it's a time when you realise . . . well a good part of your life is over, and you're now facing a time when you're on the downhill, so to speak.
> EVELYN (45–49): Sadness. Everybody seems to be tired and sad and . . . anticipating every sort of fear. Reading magazines, *Women's Weekly*s and that. . .
> CELIA (55–59): Oh, a woman whose kids have left home and is miserable and anxious and nagging and all those things. All those stereotypes that one hears about.

Celia is portraying what is commonly referred to as the 'empty nest syndrome'. However, only two women in this study regretted their children leaving home. Victoria, in her late fifties, simply responded to the question about the term 'midlife' with the word 'uncertainty', while Helena, Lenore and Renata tended to see both negative and positive dimensions to midlife. For many, strategies to control the negatives of midlife changes focused on personal health management:

> HELENA (35–39): . . . Oh, just probably. . . just getting older. . . things starting to go wrong with your body perhaps . . . and your children growing up.
> LENORE (45–49): I suppose, getting a bit older [laugh], although I have found that getting a bit older is . . . not as traumatic as it maybe could have been. I mean, in some ways, I think I'm a lot more confident,

relaxed, at ease with [my]self now, than I might have been fifteen, twenty years ago . . . and so far, my health isn't cracking up, so that's not a problem.

RENATA (40–44): I don't think of anything particularly awful, in fact I feel quite positive images. You know, I think it's a good time of your life, but I do think it's a time when you do start having to think about health care. Like, I don't have private insurance and just lately I have been thinking, you know, up ahead I'm going to have to think about it because I've not really . . . paid much attention to my health and I'm starting to think now that I'll have to.

The negative cultural representations of midlife and the uncertainty of what might be in store was depicted as more threatening by those who did not yet see themselves as entering midlife, or those who regarded themselves as being in the early stages. However, uncertainty offered both constraints and possibilities and for a minority it was a time for reflection on one's own life achievements and aspirations — a time for personal growth:

NATASHA (40–44): I think it's intensely exciting, in one sense, and fairly terrifying as well, because if you are taking leaps into something which is unknown [. . .] I certainly alternate between those two feelings.
JUDY (45–49): It's thoughtful time, I think a thoughtful time for me. I've possibly made some decisions because I have felt that it was a midlife stage and 50 is perhaps a time where you do think — well do I go on doing what I've been doing or will I aim for something different . . . possibly there is that scary aspect of how much longer do you have? Do you have another fifty, no, you think, you don't have another fifty, so [laugh] you might think about it in those terms.
MARTINE (45–49): This decade, 40 to 50, has been very, very hard, and very traumatic, but it has been just incredible in terms of my growth, in terms of . . . just getting out there and being alive, living.
ANGELA (50–54): Grown-up children and more freedom, and a second lease on life. It's quite an exciting time. I've personally found it that way, anyway. But I've always felt that your life comes in phases and this is another phase.

Thus, when asked, 'What does midlife mean?', the women responded in terms of changes to the family structure, relationships, and life expectation, while peppering their responses with an array of symptoms that included various aches and pains, as well as mental and physical changes that meshed with the chronology of social and psycho-emotional changes occurring in and around midlife.

Robyn, who is almost 40, reports that although she has not yet entered what she regards as midlife she nevertheless has increasing symptoms that are problematic. She speaks of 'stomach problems' and difficulties with her memory, which she attributes to stresses experienced at this stage of her life. Changes to well-being and body functioning are often first experienced and reported around this stage of life although they may or may not be described as 'midlife health risks'. The women were asked about various strategies they might have taken to control changes in their health, including treatment to gain symptom relief:

> ROBYN: I've read magazines about different things because I like to see what's going on but, I think I would go pretty much for tradition. I'm not one of these people that would go to the Laboyer method just to say I've gone through it. I go for my comfort, I haven't got time to do these things . . . 'Mind over matter' is something that my mother's certainly instilled in me. I think sometimes it's 'mind over matter' and that I've pushed it onto my stomach but I think a strong mind has got a lot to do with it as well, but I'll have no hesitation if those things don't work, I'll be up [to the doctor] to get the latest thing.

Robyn's collage of midlife has arisen largely from her observations of her mother and grandmother. Her mother taught her that managing much of life's experiences was a case of 'mind over matter'. She presents herself as harbouring fragments of body and mind changes handed down to her through her maternal genealogy. She reads avidly yet selectively discards segments of media propaganda on what constitutes a healthy and youthful woman's body and mind during the ageing process. She is ready to avail herself of the armoury of modern science to fend off physiological changes while embracing the contradictions of whether the maternal 'mind over matter' injunction should be part of a healthy approach to coping and managing (mid)life or whether it lends itself to a malignant oppression of body and soul. She relates her stomach problems to the stoicism demanded of herself in following her mother's adage. For her, 'mind over matter' means she seldom discusses her troubles with her husband or others yet she suspects this aggravates the troubles she is facing at this time in her life.

MIDLIFE HEALTH RISKS AS NATURAL AND UNNATURAL RISKS

Having raised the question of midlife risks, the interviewers then sought the women's views on any health risks they believed were associated with midlife.

FAMILY HISTORY AS NATURAL RISK

One hundred and twenty-nine women spoke of the family medical history of disease affecting a person's health, a further 10 said it 'probably' did, 5 said they did not know and only 16 said they did not think family history had any effect. A number of the women commented that a knowledge of family medical history influenced anxiety, attitudes, lifestyle choices, screening behaviour and other health-management activities.

The women's responses reflected the monocultural beliefs of biomedicine where people no longer die of old age, rather they die of a particular disease. It was not long before it became apparent that the majority of women regarded familial diseases as inherited risks — risks that one could do little to prevent being unleashed as a person aged. They were risks bestowed by nature and therefore were natural risks:

> PENNY (40–44): Health risk, something that . . . it's in the family and it could be passed [on] to myself or my daughter I guess, I don't know.
> CAMILLE: I guess being ignorant about your body is a health risk, for women especially, because we have a more complicated machine, don't we? . . . Well statistics show that if you've got a genetic bad heritage, that's when it comes out, in your midlife. From 40 right through.
> MEG (40–44): A health risk, well, I'd say if my grandmother and my

mother had breast cancer I would be [at] risk of getting breast cancer, that's what I would understand by it.
RHONDA (45–49): Health risk, yes. Do you mean health risk in as much as what I might have inherited from my family?

Angela, Meg and Errol are women who look to their mothers and maternal line to define their own natural risks:

> ANGELA: I'm worried about the heart disease because my mother had the bypass . . . osteoporosis . . . I'd hate that to happen. So I go and have a bone-density scan . . . I'm really worried about that because I dislike milk and I have black tea and black coffee and . . . I have cereal every second day to try and get myself a glass a milk, but I do take calcium, so . . . those two I'd say, and I'm aware of having a mammogram for breast cancer and also the Pap smears. I do all I can to prevent it.
> MEG: I think somebody told me once that Alzheimer's skips one generation and gets the next. So I always think . . . because my granny has it. But as my husband says, with Alzheimer's you're always meeting new people every day! So from the point of view that if I got it, it probably wouldn't be too bad for me, it's just everybody else around me.
> ERROL (45–49): I think I will experience some problem with my wrist and varicose veins, I have my mother's varicose veins. So I expect . . . I don't have them badly now but they probably will become bad enough for some surgical procedure later. I think that's all I expect.

Robyn had mentioned a family history of breast cancer and was determined to fight the onset of breast cancer if she could. She looked to her mother as an exemplar of resistance to disease, of mental fortitude that could protect the body from a slumbering malignancy. Yet her story suggests she felt she was not as mentally disciplined as her mother:

> Yeah, I'm not going to accept it. I try to follow my mum's lead, then if it does occur then I know that I've given it a good shot. I'm also not going to go, 'oh well', and leave it go. I've seen people that have had breasts removed that you wouldn't know unless you were told, because they have adjusted their life, it has been a hiccup, it hasn't been a catastrophe. Their attitude, their relationships, they've had to work on it, perhaps later with a bit of guidance but, they've just gone on. They've had a hiccup and off they go, so I'd like to think that I'd be like that and I think with my mum, the way she is, my husband's

support . . . I mean we've found a few hiccups and I have had scares and in the meantime, before getting tested for it, or waiting for the tests to come back, I've said to my husband, 'Well what if?' and we've sort of had good talks about it so I think I . . . I've had a lump, well I've had what I thought was a lump. I've gone up and the doctor said 'Fine, well we'll go and have it tested.' I've got breasts that are very lumpy anyway. I'm one of these women, I test myself when I'm supposed to but I find a million and I think 'Oh, God!' [Resigned tone] So I just go up to the doctor and say 'Okay, well you do it!'

These natural risks were distinguished from a second type of risk, which comprised self-inflicted behaviours such as smoking, overeating, and insufficient exercise, as well as those signs and symptoms not in themselves fatal and mostly associated with menopause.

Personal behaviour as unnatural risk

CHERYL (40–44): I guess health risk, in terms of people who smoke would have health risks as far as being more likely to develop lung cancer and so on.
CYNTHIA (35–39): Osteoporosis yes, it's probably because my mum has it, but I think that's a dietary problem because she hates milk.
VERONIKA (45–49): Osteoporosis is a thing that worries me . . . probably years ago you didn't hear so much of these things, and you didn't pick up every magazine and read something about it, and everyone is different. Just the fact that, do we eat enough of, do we have enough calcium and iron and so forth in our bodies? Do we get enough intake and all this to prevent this? As I said before, do we need the hormone treatment?

The current media concentration on women's reproductive organs and cancer and the imagery of the 'dowager's hump' of osteoporosis was reflected in the majority of women's concerns about where personal health risks lay in midlife:

LOUISE (45–49): Health risks during my midlife. Well I suppose any of the . . . ones that are considered, you know, on the statistics . . . probably osteoporosis or . . . cervical cancer.

Louise is influenced by her reading of the women's magazines and other media sources. She has noted the 'statistics' on disease probabilities, applies these to herself and is concerned. The enormous gap between such epidemiological statistics and individual clinical probabilities is not relayed through the public health messages and therefore is not reflected in the women's narratives of risk.

Tamara and Cynthia have similar assessments of their risk, which they each see as being from cancer. Tamara expresses her risks in terms of diseases that are 'around', as if their prevalence means they can be transmitted like an infectious disease:

> INTERVIEWER: You said earlier that you see yourself in midlife as being at risk of cervical and breast cancer. Why do you say that?
>
> TAMARA: I think only because it's around. You know, when you get to a certain age group, you are more at risk, you should have all these tests . . .
>
> CYNTHIA: I suppose like every woman I think of breast cancer as a big boogie, cervical cancer there's no history of it, no likelihood of that, there's no genital warts or anything that could even . . . predispose me to it.

Several of the women described managing health risks with 'healthy living' and taking medications, such as HRT, to prevent disease. Both were considered as possible means to control the unnatural risks, those that could be avoided, unlike the inherited diseases nature passed down through familial lines. While many of the women described their health strategies with their mothers and partners they most often discussed them with women friends. Ilona, aged in her late forties, was one of the women who spoke of discussing health-management strategies with friends:

> . . . and osteoporosis of course, we're all very aware of that so we worry about [it] . . . drink our skim milk and walk miles and, you know, think we're protecting ourselves from bone problems. And we talk about it.

Health risks were distinguished through three main discourses: one generated by mothers and friends (and occasionally one's partner); another by the media on the importance of diet, exercise and HRT; and the last (also reflected through the media) by the medical profession regarding the epidemiological significance of family history.

The other dimension to these health risks were those symptoms arising in association with menopause (headaches, sweats, hot flushes, sleeplessness, abnormal bleeding and cognitive changes), for which modern medicine had provided HRT as therapeutic control.

HRT TO CONTROL UNNATURAL RISKS

Forty of the women had already been taking HRT for some time to combat what has come to be no longer regarded as a natural risk. This 'unnatural' risk is one that affects all women and although 48% of the women were under 45 years at the time of the study, a quarter of the women had been treated for the 'unnatural' changes in the midlife body. HRT is promoted as a way to routinely avoid unnecessary risks or hazards of midlife. The message is, nature is unfair and the symptoms of midlife menopause are unnatural in that they are inappropriate for modern life; inappropriate and irritating. Of those who were on HRT at the time of the study, 4 had been taking it for under six months, 9 for six to twelve months, 11 for one to four years and 5 for five to ten years. None had been on it longer than ten years. Twenty-seven of the women who were not on HRT expressed certainty that they would take it to relieve symptoms when they occurred and a further 16 said they would consider taking HRT if symptoms became disabling. Seven said they probably would not take it and 9 said they definitely would not. A further 11 said they had not yet thought about it. These statistics reflect increasing market constructions of need influencing women in this society. In the late 1980s it was believed only around 20% of women would be on HRT (Ballinger & Walker 1987).

In this study, HRT was largely unrelated to screening or prevention. The strongest association for the women between HRT and midlife was symptom control, that is, as treatment. Only 12 women talked about HRT as a possible preventative, eight of these were voiced as doctor-initiated discussions where the doctor promoted the use of HRT to prevent a disease:

> INTERVIEWER: So the hormone replacement therapy for this, you'd be likely to consider . . .
> ROBYN: Yes.
> INTERVIEWER: What symptoms would you need to have to consider that?
> ROBYN: Things that would really interfere with my lifestyle. Hot flushes are one. I've seen people, they've been people who've had hot flushes and they've just said it was almost like a tingle, just a hot tingle. I've worked with a lady who was absolutely saturated and I think that I wouldn't put up with that, I wouldn't because I can see me working for quite a few years and if I happen to hit menopause while I [am] still working and it was interfering with my lifestyle in a radical way . . . yeah, I'd hit the hormone therapy, the exercise, in a big way. I'd really go hammer and tongs to decrease those symptoms.

The majority of the women who were under 55 years of age saw these as health risks foreshadowing diseases that a person could take action to prevent (or at least control). Women could exercise, consume a healthy diet and undertake other interventions, including HRT. As symptoms, these midlife risks were mostly irritating and although nature imposed obstacles to a smooth transition through the ageing process the effects were controllable. These women had absorbed the messages of individual responsibility imposed through health promotion messages. Sociocultural or sociodemographic contributing factors did not enter the women's explanations of accountability. These health risks were mostly the fault of the individual as these were avoidable and unnecessary.

This is entirely consistent with the biomedical view that such unnecessary symptoms result from one of nature's misdemeanours. The basis of this view is that nature has not yet adapted to the social manipulations of public health and clinical medicine that ensure a longevity whereby people no longer die in their thirties or forties when such symptoms would have marked the natural desiccation of the human body. Menopausal symptoms now demarcating midlife instead of the termination of life have become an anomaly of nature. These symptoms can be seen as an anachronism, as unnatural.

While the women's stories did not go so far as to spell out the history of medicine and its oft-depicted views of the midlife anomaly, their stories nevertheless cast inherited or familial health risks as having a strong measure of inevitability as natural risks, while the risks of smoking, failing to consume calcium-rich dairy foods, not undertaking enough exercise, as well as the lack of control of the symptoms of menopause, were distinctly seen as being one's own fault, a personal choice, self-imposed health risks that were unnatural risks the individual chose to impose on the body.

SCREENING TO PREDICT DISEASE

Screening is undertaken widely in Australian society, the theory underpinning the practice being that indicators of disease ('risk factors') will be revealed through the screening process and will act as predictors for a particular disease. A further assumption is that it is the individual's responsibility to embark on a disease-prevention program should such 'risk factors' be identified. In short, it is widely believed that to predict 'risk factors' is to prevent disease. In addition, although screening practices might be promoted through a rhetoric of health and advocated as an activity promoting a healthy lifestyle, they are, nevertheless, disease-model focused.

Screening is largely a gendered surveillance activity, aspects of which are promoted as being necessary for women from their twenties (for example, the Pap smear test). We therefore asked the women if, in relation to perceived health risks associated with midlife, they underwent screening for particular diseases and to what end.

Only 6 women in the study (3.6%) had never undergone any screening in their lives (the concept being defined by the interviewer following initial questions, in order to gain valid responses). One hundred and forty-nine women (89%) had undergone at least one Pap smear test and 43 women (26%) were having Pap smears conducted annually (despite medical recommendations that Pap smears need be conducted only once every two years). Forty-eight (29%) had this test two-yearly, 35 (21%) were having them at other intervals, 4 (2.4%) were having them more often than annually due to existing pathology.

The majority of the women believed that screening would somehow prevent them developing the particular condition for which they were being tested:

> LIV (45–49): I think I am facing probably all of those [heart disease, cancer, Alzheimer's, severe arthritis], I mean there's a possibility, er . . . no that's silly . . . because I assume I'm not going to have breast cancer or uterine cancer because I have regular checks and things.

Liv articulates a significant feature of many of the women's stories. There was a frequently held belief that 'to be screened is to prevent disease occurrence' for that disease. This is an important observation for those promoting health and screening behaviours as it is an inaccurate belief. Monique (aged 60) has a Pap smear to 'avoid getting cancer or [to have] it detected early'. However, there were also statements, such as Abigail's (aged 55–59), that 'the doctor' had given assurances that having a Pap smear would 'prevent cervical cancer 100%', although Abigail did not believe this. Only a few women stated that they did not believe that screening would prevent the disease. Nevertheless, it was still widely believed that screening would prevent the disease from being either serious or fatal. Fifty-six of the women said they hoped to gain early intervention in the disease process should pathology be noted, while 45 of the women said they underwent health screening for 'security' or 'peace of mind'. This confirms the influence of health promotion messages that correlate health screening with disease prevention or disease control. This is significant as such a correlation is somewhat more tenuous when one examines the scientific literature on true outcomes of screening (Parsons & Buckenham 1991).

While women had absorbed health promotion messages, some revealed a varied logic in terms of their perceptions of personal health risk. If we return for a moment to the vignette at the start of this chapter we see a woman, Susan, who believes the odds of developing cancer are minimal, firstly because she undergoes frequent screening which she believes will insulate her from cervical cancer and, secondly, because so many women around her have had breast cancer she feels this alters her statistical probability of acquiring breast disease. The excerpt is interesting as it is about risk probabilities, and about partial understanding and selective understanding of the association between health risk and screening. The contradiction in her concatenation of fact and fiction seems born of a fear of the condition, more than reasoned risk assessment.

The routinisation of health screening

What were the women's experiences of screening and how did their experiences affect their screening behaviour? Experiences of screening were varied. Many of the women spoke of embarrassment and had tried to routinise, or make ordinary, what are often extraordinary procedures:

> SHONA (60): Just a procedure, not a five minute procedure that is of no consequence [however] it doesn't take any time. If I have an ordinary appointment, I get my blood pressure checked and Pap smear and I'm out the door.

None of the women liked having breast or cervical screening and many reported getting it over and done with as quickly as possible, not wanting to know more about the procedures or the test results. Many said they did not follow up their test results and assumed if there was anything wrong with the result then the doctor would contact them. While most women undertook screening for cervical and breast cancer as routine, forty-three women reported avoiding screening in general and gave a rationale for why they did not access screening regularly or at all. Some were 'too frightened', some believed it was 'not necessary', some were 'too embarrassed', others 'did not want to know' the results. Yet others had negative experiences that strongly influenced their screening behaviour:

> ELEANOR [speaking of her first experience of mammography]: No, I was horrified about it [laughing] it was really a plonk! And it was Ugh! [laughing] It was sort of a bit barbaric.
>
> MARION (45–49) [who had previously had one mammogram without a problem]: On the second occasion . . . I went to a different place and I really didn't like their approach and it was different. To the point where my breasts were squeezed paper thin, in between two plates . . . I found that very off-putting. It was uncomfortable. It was painful. It was certainly most uncomfortable, and unpleasant. In fact I haven't been back since then.
>
> INTERVIEWER: It's been a deterrent.
>
> MARION: It has in some respects, although I know that I ought to go back and I shall go back . . .
>
> RHONDA: Yes, I wouldn't say I've had good experiences. I remember I would have only been about 29, and I hadn't had a Pap smear for a couple of years, and I remember thinking 'it's time I went' . . . and he [the doctor] scrambled around in the cupboards again, and finally he got out the silver thing [cervical speculum] can't think of the name of it, and he inserted it, and then he said 'Oh, can you hang on to this for a minute, I forgot the slide.' So, there I was, lying up there on the table, staring at this speck on the wall thinking 'I can't believe this is happening to me.' He didn't want to do it, now I've got to hang on to it, there I am lying there hanging on to this silver thing, while he scrounges around in his cupboard . . . The last one I had was very painful, from this female doctor. It's never hurt me before. But the last one I had was enough to make me not ever want to go back again. It hurt me so badly. First of all . . . it was the wrong size she said . . . so, she had to take it out again, and off she went and found another one and came back and inserted that. I remember even as she was adjusting it, I could hear her adjusting it, and already it was beginning to hurt and I thought, 'This is strange, it's never hurt me before.' She was very rough, very rough. And, afterwards I thought, 'Well I'm not going back to her for one again either so . . . '

Women are being given advice from their doctors to undergo Pap smears, as a routine from the time they become sexually active. For some, this means beginning in their teens:

PENNY: I had it done because he [the doctor] said it was a good idea. But I really didn't think . . . I thought I was far too young. Now I go along routinely because I'm getting to the age where I think it could be a problem. At 20 you don't appreciate what things could happen to you later on in life.

INTERVIEWER: Your Pap smears, how long were you having those before your hysterectomy?
NORA (50–54): Oh, I feel I've always had one. I used to go to the gynaecologist, I think regularly. I can't recall if I went every year but that was a routine procedure.

When so many of the women underwent health screening, often on a regular basis, it must be recognised that this is not a mundane activity however 'routine' it may become. These are women who have subjected their own bodies to medical surveillance, sometimes to most intimate and invasive procedures. These women subjected themselves to screening partly because of a perceived disease threat and partly because they trusted the health messages they were hearing.

DISEASE THREAT AS MOTIVATION FOR SCREENING

Consistent with the belief that everyone dies of a disease rather than old age, of the 167 women asked 'Do you think there is a particular disease that you believe you will get at any stage in your life?', 82 women (49%) said 'yes'. When asked to name the disease their responses ranked as follows (the women could nominate more than one disease): cancer 27.8% (breast cancer 14%, uterine cancer 6.6%, colon cancer 1.8%, other specific cancers 4.2%, cancer in general 1.2%); heart disease 16%; and osteoporosis 14%. Only a third of the women (29%) said 'no', while others had not previously thought about such a question. As 78% of the women had said 'yes' or 'no' we wanted to know what the remainder had said. These clustered into two main responses: 'hadn't thought about it' and 'didn't know'. Seventeen had to be rated as non-responders.

This profile of women's beliefs about their personal susceptibility reflects media reporting of epidemiological data rather than real projections of individual morbidity or mortality. Of the women who said they did not think they would get a particular disease, a few felt they were susceptible to several illnesses, mainly attributable to family medical history or prior personal illness, while some thought they were going to be able to avoid or delay morbidity in midlife.

There is little doubt that for all the variations in responses, the women in this study had absorbed the health promotion messages of biomedicine and its media outlets. This information was being translated by the majority of women into a bodily self-discipline. Reading the interview transcripts and comparing responses to questions about the physical and mental dimensions of daily life gives the reader a sense of the hustle and bustle of bodily enhancements but little sense of well-being, of satisfaction with the hand that life had dealt each woman.

Trusting self, public health messages and healers

Generally, the interviews reveal the sense of power and control that women feel they have over their own bodies, although they appear to have little over their life circumstances, or life risks. For all that the logic in women's narratives varied and contradictions could be identified (as is normal in everyday speech); in general, the women portrayed a common picture of knowing their own bodies and trusting their own predictions associated with health risks. Their narratives are of women reading their bodies and trusting their own judgments in the light of available public information and family medical histories. From the selections they make, they construct their personal collages of midlife risks and strategies for control.

There is also an overall trust of healers woven through these narratives, whether the healer is trained in allopathic medicine or naturopathic healing. Robyn's discussion of her mother's breast disease and her own risk of breast cancer generated discussion around her trust of her healer:

> INTERVIEWER: And you trust the messages that they're giving you, the information they're giving you?
> ROBYN: Yes, I do. I don't blindly have faith in this guy [her doctor] . . . I do have trust in him . . . the fact that if I need a kick in the backside that's all I get, he's not a prescription writer for the sake of it. If he thinks that . . . he can't help me, he will refer me . . . yes I do trust him. He's someone that I can really talk to and he will answer you and it doesn't matter if there's a waiting-room full of people, you know . . . he looks after your mental health as well.

Robyn provides the criteria of a trustworthy doctor, 'the fact that if I need a kick in the backside', 'he's not a prescription writer for the sake of it', if 'he can't help me, he will refer me', and perhaps most importantly, 'he's someone that I can really talk to'. And there is more:

> INTERVIEWER: . . . you're very fortunate aren't you.
> ROBYN: Oh he's lovely, I said if you ever shift I'm following you . . . yes, I do trust him but if there was . . . a time when I thought, no, that just doesn't sound right, or I wasn't happy, I would go somewhere else but I've never got to that stage because he does supply all the information and he does help.

This woman, with a family history of breast disease and with a mother as a mentor whom she relies on for guidance in health care, also steeped herself in other health risk discourses making her selections of what she regarded as relevant snippets of knowledge to add to her collage of midlife and health-risk.

Deni (in her early forties), although young, has previously experienced the threat of cancer. She believes that careful medical monitoring will prevent recurrence. She shares the trust in her medical carers that many women expressed:

> The cancer risk, well, sure there is a risk that perhaps in the next five years I may have another lump in my other breast but I'm not particularly worried because of the care and help that I'm getting, so other than that, I don't feel any other current risks.

Interestingly, although Beryl (in her late thirties) is one of the few women who reported choosing to see alternative healers, the women who did so were mostly concerned about different diseases from those promoted and given emphasis in biomedical public health policy:

> I know for a fact, with myself, my pancreas . . . I've been to naturopaths and natural healing where they look into your eyes and they can tell what parts of your body aren't functioning properly. And, I've been told that my pancreas isn't working properly or something like that, therefore the foods that I'm taking into myself aren't necessarily being fully used. And, also the wastes from that food aren't being pushed through and out properly, so that's my danger.

Liv describes herself as being 'into natural healing':

> Herbs, yes. Rather than take a tablet I lie down and meditate . . . It's not full natural healing . . . I'll go to a naturopath rather than go to a GP, not that I don't believe in them, I do, but I believe that if a naturopath can't cure me, then I will go to a GP.

However, trust is discretionary and a number of the women were sceptical of various discourses, especially those from the media. The women were of an age to have sufficient confidence and maturity to ask their own questions of their life trajectories and make their own decisions regarding their perceived risks. They read and listened to the health and disease messages, identifying the source (the legitimacy of the message and the messenger) and assessed both. They were consumers of various discourses on health and illness, evaluated such knowledge, several expressing some disdain at the hyperbole of media messages:

> SUSAN: What sort of health messages would get my attention? Oh, look, I don't think much would because there's so much being pushed at you all the time that nothing's sensational any more.
> ANGELA: I feel [there's] almost too much made of it at the moment. But if any good is going to come of anything, it usually has to be exaggerated and go to extremes first before everybody will accept it and it will calm down and go back to it's correct perspective.

In sum, much of the discussion generated by the women about family risks was couched in terms of the natural inheritance of particular diseases. Carried by nature, this natural risk was virtually unavoidable. The women's voices reflected medical discourses on risks as inherited and passed on by nature in family genetics, as well as risk from oestrogen deficiency which was an unnecessary harbinger of midlife disorder. How one fared in midlife was largely under the control of the individual with the aid of medicine and its allies. This is consistent with the fact that few of the women took HRT as a disease preventative. Rather, most took it to alleviate symptoms (treatment for the deficiency that was menopause), which were regarded as something to be controlled or avoided as unnecessary, unnatural and unacceptable. Where nature had failed to do her part, medicine could offer a reprieve from nature's vagaries and assist her to make the necessary adjustments to the reality of a longer average lifespan.

There are implications here for both health promotion campaigns and the media: more accurate reporting of the links between epidemiological data and individual clinical outcomes is required, and the level of anxiety and guilt generated through health messages about screening and the effects that lifestyle has on disease outcomes should be examined. It is also clear that improved medical education would benefit some in the medical profession who conduct health screening, making it a more positive experience for women, especially as they are induced to continue screening for over half of their lives.

9
WHAT *DID* THE DOCTOR SAY?

Lyn Richards

JESS: I've sort of got to the point now where I've read so much literature that I've got myself completely bamboozled. And, I keep thinking, and arguing with myself, because part of me would like very much to take this pill that they tell me I can take and stay looking lovely and beautiful like they tell me I'm going to. My doctor said to me, 'Mother Nature has made a mistake. Mother Nature isn't always right.' And, I thought, 'Wait a minute.' And, he said, 'Of course, she can't correct it because the breeding cycle of humans is finished, so we've got to do it for her. That's why you need HRT. You'll feel so much better. Your skin won't get wrinkly, you won't get heart disease, you won't get osteoporosis. You'll be wonderful.' And I said 'Oh, is there any guarantee that I'm going to get osteoporosis if I don't take it anyway? And, will I necessarily get heart disease if I don't take it?' He couldn't give me . . . I said, 'OK, what [are] the negatives?' 'There aren't any.' I said, 'What about cancer?' 'It's not related to cancer.' Yet all the reading I've done says very strongly that it is . . . Then in the next breath he said to me some of the studies have shown a slight increase in breast cancer. 'Slight very slight. Nothing to worry about.' But then the studies, from what I've seen, are only for five years, which doesn't really tell you anything. I mean, five years from now, if I took nothing, I would probably still be alright. And, if I took something, I would probably be alright . . .

LYN: So, you walked out without oestrogen?

JESS: I did. His parting comment to me was 'I'll get you on it if it's the last thing I do, because the only "anti" things that you could hear would be that it's not natural.'

So far, this book has told women's stories of their experiences and how they interpreted them. But the women's voices are backed by other voices, which offer other, sometimes rival, accounts of the menopause from those who 'claim rights as interpreters to women of their bodies' experiences' (Kaufert 1982, p. 141). In what women read or learned and how they interpreted it there often appeared one or both of two competing interpretations, from the medical profession and from the community health level. This chapter and the next are about these other voices offering health advice. This chapter is concerned with the messages of the medical profession and, in particular, that segment most consulted by women about menopause — general practitioners. Chapter 10 focuses on health care at the 'grass roots' community level, where women's health messages are heard much more clearly and are at least sometimes combined with opposition to the 'biomedical perspective'.

If any of us was tempted to the assumption that doctors' advice is homogeneous and known, we were rapidly forced to jettison it. In doing so, we were brought up against strong assumptions in the popular and sociological literature that women seeking health advice confront a hostile 'biomedical perspective'. As shown in the previous chapters, women's reports of doctors' advice were far more varied than either the sociological or the popular literature led us to expect.

Some, but by no means all, fitted splendidly the critical image of blind biomedical interpretation. Each of us has interviewed at least one woman who, like Jess, says her doctor said things that are clearly patriarchal, insensitive, treatment-oriented and/or just plain false. These quotes, taken out of context, make great cinema. Of course we don't know what Jess's doctor did say. But every such story seems to confirm the ugly image of the 'biomedical perspective'. And women's language often suggests that they accept medical authority unquestioningly.

As the project proceeded, we discovered the complicated results of not assuming we know in advance what the doctor said (or indeed what any other health provider said). Women's accounts could be fitted into a model of a single biomedical perspective only if we refused to accept a high proportion of their stories. Certainly we had striking stories, like Jess's, of doctors' apparently dogmatic assertion of medical solutions. As the critical literature led us to expect these, they tended to dominate our early picture of the data. However we often seemed to have as many stories of doctors' concerns at their own lack of information, or explicit advice against medical solutions, contradicting the stereotype.

In search of the 'biomedical perspective'

Assertions about the biomedical perspective/model/bias or view are rarely accompanied by evidence. When evidence is reported, it is most commonly from reviews of usually old medical texts, which are splendid sources of hilarious quotations. A review of medical literature from the 1960s led Logothetis (1991, p. 40) to conclude:

> The menopausal woman seems to elicit a particularly virulent brand of negativity on the part of physicians. She has been depicted as being no longer attractive or sexually desirable, as being no longer needed, and as a degraded outcast no longer capable of achievement. In short, she has been portrayed as experiencing her menopause as a process of decay rather than development.

However, the possibility that not all of today's doctors unquestioningly believe or act upon the brief and unattractive depictions of women in past textbooks is rarely explored. Lock (1982, p. 263) points out that there is an assumption in much recent social science writing about menopause that 'a shared medical model is adhered to rather closely by clinicians' and moreover that 'contents of texts for medical and lay audiences are closely allied to, or even synonymous with, ideas and behaviour that patients will encounter in a clinical setting'.

There are problems with beginning from the assertion that there is a dominant model of scientific medicine creating sick and docile individuals. It is easy to set up research to prove the existence of straightforward, gross medical power. There are predictable places where women's experiences and bodies are seen as entirely understandable in terms of biomedical process, with particular emphasis, in this context, on hormones and, inevitably, socially undesirable ageing. We have known for some time that medical texts grossly distort women's experience (Kaufert 1982). An early sector of our project did conduct a review of past medical texts, and this exercise, not surprisingly, found a consistently negative 'biomedical' interpretation, albeit a markedly changing one (Daly, Miller & Richards 1992). However, we knew little about the extent to which the knowledge provided in texts was accepted by the people who practised medicine, and the ways this or other knowledge was conveyed by them to women, let alone what women did with it. And the possibilities of other knowledge and processes of interpretation of it remained unexplored.

Several major issues arise here. Firstly, should we predict from such data to behaviour? How and by what processes are those texts interpreted — if they are even known?

Secondly, whatever the relevance of texts to clinical behaviour in general, menopause is likely to be an area in which that relevance is minimised. Knowledge of menopause is highly disputed, increasing and changing rapidly, popularly available, heavily promoted and noisily debated in the popular media. Medical texts, by contrast, have very little to say about menopause, although they have a lot to say on the larger question of hormones and women's bodies. This is not to argue that it is irrelevant to review medical textbooks. Doing so established one of the many threads possibly contributing to doctor's knowledge and behaviour. We do, however, know that medical texts use the language of medical textbooks, a fact that is hardly surprising.

To start with the assertion of dominance, and deduce explanations from it, is to resort to what Michel Foucault (probably the most cited writer asserting medical dominance) called a 'descending type of analysis, the one of which I believe one ought to be wary':

> One can always make this deduction, it is always easily done and that is precisely what I would hold against it . . . These kinds of deduction

are always possible. They are simultaneously correct and false. Above all they are too glib. (1977, p. 100)

Foucault urged 'an ascending analysis of power, starting, that is, from its infinitesimal mechanisms', and looking for 'the forms of resistance against different forms of power' (1977, p. 780).

One way of doing this would be to listen to the stories of health advisers about their interactions with women. If we really want to know how and what doctors contribute to women's understanding of menopause, it just won't do to assume they act from the text of a book they may never have read or, if they have read it, have probably forgotten, as it occupied a tiny part of their training and is now out of date. That probably-forgotten unread text has even less relevance if it did not say anything about the issues raised by the experience of the woman in front of them. We need accounts from the doctors of what they think they know, and how they see their clinical interactions.[1]

WHAT DO CRITICS SAY DOCTORS SAY?

Few researchers have actually asked the doctors what they say to women about menopause. Far more have asked the medical texts. Lock (1982) did both, conducting a literature review of texts and an interview and observation study. She found an almost complete variety of approach to the topic and the women: variety in the amount of background information, seeking of symptoms, interpretation of them, willingness to nominate oestrogen treatment, and perception and presentation of arguments for and against it. She argued it was important 'to make a clear distinction between textual knowledge and practice . . . Individual physicians are inclined to work from folk models which form the basis for their decision-making. The contents of the folk models are very rich and subject to constant modification' (p. 277).

The so-called 'biomedical perspective' as portrayed in critical accounts is not only subject to modification but has many faces, so it is hard to weigh what doctors say against this amorphous model. However its various depictions seem to have a common set of key features, summarised in Figure 9.1. Each, or at least most, of the critics make some of the following linked claims: that doctors have a special type of attitude to care, of relationship to women patients, of 'scientific' knowledge, and, behind all this, of power.

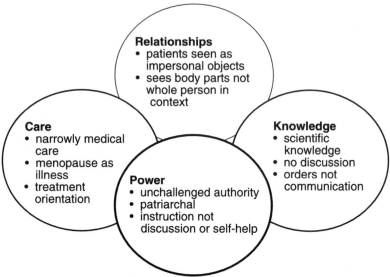

Figure 9.1 Themes in the critical stereotype of the 'biomedical model'.

CARE

Doctors are said to emphasise 'medicalisation' of the social or personal. Menopause is interpreted as a deficiency disease, with a degrading emphasis on women's physical deterioration and on treatment, and rejection of any 'natural' therapy or 'alternative' cures. In the context of menopause, the 'medical model' is said to look only at the positives of HRT, denying or even lying about the negatives. MacPherson's 15-year-old attack is still widely quoted:

> Patriarchal, misogynous gynaecologists and psychiatrists officially directed and profited from the transformation of menopause into a disease while women who experienced it have rarely discussed it in any detail, even among themselves. This myth of menopause as disease

has been so successfully marketed to the American public that currently most women associate the word menopause with depression if not mental illness, osteoporosis if not cancer. Because menopause has been labelled a disease, women believe they must be 'treated' by physicians with carcinogenic estrogens in order to be 'cured'. (1981, p. 96)

Relationships

In the biomedical model this is supposed to be an impersonal and object-oriented interaction, with the emphasis on time and cost of interaction. Patriarchal definitions of women's purposes and roles are believed to predominate, providing a stereotypic picture of the menopausal woman as irritable, frequently depressed, asexual, and besieged by hot flushes:

> The extant knowledge of menopause transmits and perpetuates, through the sanctity of science and the authority of the medical 'expert', the knowledge and power relations that help structure and reinforce society's expectations and stereotypes of menopausal women. These stereotypes and myths impose restricted positions on women as they are classified as products of their reproductive systems and hormones. (Dickson 1990, pp. 16–17)

Knowledge

The contention is that the importance, reliability and validity of 'scientific knowledge' is very narrowly defined, and excludes individual understanding. The 'narrow' focus on the physical symptoms and biological changes leads to an overlooking of social transitions and strategies. This sort of knowledge is said to ignore experience and context.

Power

The critics discuss doctors' power, control and authority in general and, in particular, patriarchal control of women's medical experiences. Women are said to be derided and degraded in this relationship.

These are overlapping and not necessarily consistent sets of ideas. However most descriptions of the medical perspective seem to include some ingredients from each of the four value clusters. The emphasis is on power, but most of the critique is not explicitly about power. Rather, sets of ideas about power overlap only partially with sets of ideas about health care, about relationships with patients and, behind all this, about knowledge and certainty. Each of these in turn partially overlaps with the others. There seem, in fact, to be few statements in which all of these claims are being made. None of the critics are asserting that *all* doctors will show *all* of these behaviours and beliefs, rather that they fit together in what perhaps could be called a syndrome. However, the relationships between them are rarely examined.

WHAT DO THE DOCTORS SAY THEY SAID?

We took the direct approach and asked the doctors what they told women about menopause. We wrote to all general practitioners and alternative health professionals in each of our five areas, asking them to fill in a one-page questionnaire or do a face-to-face interview. Thirty accepted, and 20 of these did a taped interview. The sample is too small to report proportions and its skew is obviously towards doctors who saw women's issues as of interest or their own roles as problematic. Other things being equal, we would expect that doctors most wedded to a hard-line patriarchal, narrowly biological interpretation of menopause would be least likely to wish to spend time talking to women sociologists. Thus we have no basis in this data for assessing how common such a perspective is among doctors, or how wide the range of approaches they take.

We did, however, discover a surprisingly wide range of approaches even among our volunteer sample. The interviews showed a wide variety of information and approaches. They drew attention to the local sources of women's knowledge, and to the importance of socio-economic and demographic context, and the availability of information and services. In the following section, the data are discussed under each of the four dimensions of the biomedical stereotype.

CARE

There are three major clusters of ideas in the criticism of doctors' attitudes to care. Is it narrowly medical? Does it treat menopause as a deficiency disease? And is treatment emphasised over consultation?

NARROWLY MEDICAL?

'Medicalisation' of the social or personal is a major theme in the critique. It is also an interesting criticism. Absence of medical knowledge would, of course, be a major cause for complaint. Indeed we met that one, with women's criticisms that the doctor was asking *them* for ideas or experience. When we talked with doctors, not surprisingly, none denied medical knowledge. Several did, however, express concern at their inability to keep up to date with epidemiological research.

In this context 'narrowly medical' usually refers to unthinking or exclusive reliance on hormone treatment and lack of interest in other strategies or in the social context of women's experience. Hardly surprisingly, since we asked, all of the doctors offered or implied knowledge of the biological processes of menopause and the epidemiological status of HRT. We did not ask questions about the social changes women experience at this time, but all of them spent at least some time discussing these aspects of midlife.

One young woman doctor's views about medical care for menopause contradicted the stereotype in virtually every way:

> I think it has to be patient specific. So it relates very much to the patient and the family situation. So it is looking at the person as a whole. I mean, obviously what you are going to be focusing on at that particular age are the symptoms of menopause and the associated factors that are linked to that particular time in a woman's life... First of all I think it is important to discuss with the patient what their understanding of menopause is; what they have heard and if any of

their friends have actually experienced the menopause; what they know about it.

HRT comes up in this context, but so, she insists, do social factors:

> I mean, we haven't even talked about the other aspects of a woman's life at this particular point. You know, the kids have left school and how they are feeling and their general health. Often it will be their calcium that comes up. They should be taking calcium and [doing] weight-bearing exercises.

Asked if the safety of HRT had been established, of the twenty doctors interviewed only two were convinced that HRT was 'clearly safe'. Most ticked 'still under debate' out of four options. However all prescribed it for some women, and only two implied they would resist if a woman asked to be prescribed HRT. As one said, 'People don't come that way. They don't come and say "I want oestrogen". They come and say basically that "I hear that there are hormones that can be given after you've gone through the change. Tell me about it."'

MENOPAUSE AS A DEFICIENCY DISEASE?

The interview closest to the biomedical stereotype was with a young male doctor who had made a specialty of obstetrics and gynaecology and resented the intrusion of menopause clinics into this territory. He said the topic of HRT usually came up because women came in with symptoms, often having gained information elsewhere. He always gave them material to read, but admitted it was biased:

> Sometimes they present because of lectures or advice or written articles they have seen about HRT and they know that I'm interested in it. I do give them a booklet on the menopause with a bias towards HRT but nevertheless it's a good booklet ... And if they have got oestrogen deficiency symptoms I usually order HRT.

His was the most confident ruling on the treatment (and the terms 'deficiency' and 'ordering' occurred in no other interview):

> I see it as clearly safe. The only proviso I think is that I see young girls about 18 and we often put them on the pill which is oestrogen and

progesterone. They take that through to menopause and then we go and promptly give them the same hormones for a variable period of time . . . If they haven't had a family history of breast cancer, I find them more likely to take HRT. If there is a family history and it is strong, I certainly wouldn't push it.

This doctor took the line of Jess's general practitioner, a line we have heard from several parts of the medical system: mother nature made a mistake; women are now living into their eighties:

> So they are facing a new problem and you can't say that HRT is abnormal because it is no more abnormal than the fact that they live so long into the menopause.

Each of the doctors, not surprisingly, discussed and conducted oestrogen level tests and assessed the evidence of women's changed hormone levels. Most, when they discussed the use of such data, mentioned that it was taken in context of the women's lives.

Treatment orientation?

Only one of the doctors we interviewed recommended any treatment other than mainstream medical strategies, and all had prescribed HRT for some patients. However none, in this small group, offered the stereotyped inflexible approach that would put all women at midlife on oestrogen. The nearest is Dr Chris:

> There is no doubt it prevents the cardiovascular problems. There is also no doubt probably hormone replacement therapy on its own, but certainly in conjunction with calcium, prevents bone loss. Probably hormone replacement therapy on its own, if they have a diet that is sufficient [in] calcium, is all you need. But in conjunction with calcium there is no doubt that the two together work. Whereas there is considerable doubt about whether calcium on its own without hormone replacement therapy does any good or not. So we are preventing the cardiovascular problems. We are preventing the bone loss problems. I also have no doubts in my own mind that hormone replacement therapy for most women keeps them fitter generally. Their general health is improved. I have no doubt that their general health is better, they feel better, they look better. I think that there is no doubt that it prevents ageing of the skin and the ageing of the tissues that occurs. I am also fairly convinced that their sexual health is better as

well . . . Their sexual health is better and they feel better about themselves. They feel more attractive and I believe it prevents the ageing . . . No it doesn't prevent the ageing process but it stops women from prematurely ageing.

His ruling: clearly safe. The statement raises an interesting issue: why do doctors who rule the treatment 'clearly safe' still insist that it be the woman's decision? Dr Chris again:

I would think that there might be exceptions for particular risk groups. But otherwise as long as the woman is happy and content to be on it and I think there are still some women who would refuse it, but if after having discussed it fairly completely with the patient, if she was happy to go on it then I think she should be on it. If she was unhappy for whatever reason, I wouldn't push the issue . . . I wouldn't say 'You should be on it' or 'I'm unhappy that you are not on it.' It would be entirely up to the patient. But as long as they were happy, I would think all women should be on it except that there . . . the risk groups are not really . . . there are not many that come into the risk groups that I can think of. I would be thinking of breast cancer . . . and I suppose if there had been uterine cancer of any sort although in most cases they would have had a hysterectomy I would presume. [Otherwise] I see no reason not to put her on hormone replacement therapy.

But most doctors expressed discomfort at drug companies and the need for changing medical practice featured here. This is not a response of only women or the young. Contrast the responses of an elderly male general practitioner and a young woman:

God! To put things in balance, hormone replacement therapy has basically been the flavour of the month in the last eighteen months and I think that when [we] look at hormone replacement therapy, we've got to be very careful that we see it in its right context because . . . There has been tremendous publicity for hormone replacement therapy and it has been featured in all the women's magazines . . . After all there are a lot of women, and I can take you around tomorrow, to say, thirty women who are in their nineties and who have had good health. They didn't have hormone replacement therapy . . . We've had some statements that say 'All women over 35 should be put on HRT and anyone who doesn't put women on it is [medically] negligent.' That frightens me . . . Let's look at the bottom line. That's lovely for drug companies.

The woman general practitioner saw a process of change, in which she was an active participant:

> I think that while the medical profession see hormone replacement treatment in many cases being very positive, I think we need to step back and look at whether that is really appropriate. It is medicalising again. I do personally have some difficulties with that . . . That is why I think anything like hormone replacement therapy has to be very patient-specific. It really has to be beneficial to them . . . I think we have to get away from that sort of medicine anyway. It is not the medicine of the nineties.

Every doctor interviewed recommended HRT to some patients. Each said they would do so only after detailed investigation of symptoms. Some, but not all, expressed confidence that the recommendation was unproblematic. Most, but not all, emphasised women's being informed and making their own informed choice. A few saw it as the doctor's, not the woman's, choice.

Relationships

The second set of ideas in the biomedical stereotype fits poorly with our data. Doctor–patient relations are hotly debated in the literature, with the dominant theme being that the patient is seen as a biological blob, with emphasis on symptoms, on body parts and their malfunctions, rather than the 'whole person'. The relationship with the doctor is seen as isolating, individual, and one of instruction, not one of communication, understanding and mutual decision. If this is so, we would expect that doctors' accounts of their interactions with patients would show evidence of impersonal and object-oriented interaction, with emphasis on time and cost of interaction.

Again, of course, our data has limitations. Nobody was likely to tell us that they saw women at menopause as a bundle of hormones and malfunctioning reproductive organs, or that they refused to discuss it and pushed them out with pills as fast as possible. One male doctor said others treated menopause like diabetes, just reaching for the 'cure'. And one doctor in a rural area did imply this was true of his urban colleagues:

I think that's why I like practising in the rural areas, because you can't practise medicine unless you know what's going on with the family, it's not possible. You've just got to make it in-and-out medicine otherwise. It's like the 24-hour clinics. People come in, you don't know [who] they are, they present a throat infection, give them antibiotics, if they come in with flushes, they get oestrogen and out they go. There is no personal interaction . . .

Attention to the words used gave some clues. The discourse of some doctors suggested that interaction and discussion were not seen as central to their role (they 'put her on' HRT, or 'order' it). Nicole and Cathy noticed during coding our interview transcripts that the doctors tended to use the verb 'complain' to describe interaction: patients coming 'complaining of their symptoms'.

Two doctors in older age groups used words many women would interpret as patriarchal:

I mean many girls are peri-menopausal at 47. Some are quite well and menstrual and regular at the age of 52. So 47-year-olds might be spoken to and [for] the 52s [it] might be just suggested that when their periods stop in three to six months, we'd like to talk to them about hormone replacement therapy . . . Some girls can't take it.

We were firmly given some negative messages but these were negative towards menopause as an area of practice, not towards women:

From a doctor's point of view, when that sort of consultation is obviously about to take place and [women patients] open up a consultation saying they think they might be going through the change for this, this and this reason — I won't say my heart sinks exactly, but I often make it clear early on that any menopausal consultation is quite long, and that it involves a lot of talking and then involves a full physical examination, and then it involves discussing medication if you are going to use any so that . . . I say, 'Today I would like to just have a talk, and then I'll get you back to do the examination and the medication hormones if we need it.' People don't think. They just make an appointment and don't think that perhaps fifteen minutes isn't anywhere near long enough to cover such an enormous area.

Several doctors expressed irritation with the difficulties of arriving at the right dose or dealing with side-effects, and two at the way menopause had become 'flavour of the month'. Several were irritated by the constant updating of knowledge and seminars they had no time to attend. One male doctor made it clear his role is directive, and the main problem is clarity of instructions:

> There was a journal lobbed on my desk last week which detailed the various treatment regimes that are available . . . which I read with interest because it is messy trying to prescribe hormone replacement therapy. It is not clear and easy . . . I think it would make life easier if we had [pill packaging] where you could say 'Right, the first two weeks contain both [oestrogen and progesterone] and the next two weeks just contain the oestrogen. Start there and finish there and go on to the next box.'

This sounds very like the stereotype of biomedical care. However the same doctor, like almost all the others, gave an account that suggested considerable clinical consultation and discussion, and recognition of women's knowledge and ability to make decisions about treatment:

> I always leave the treatment . . . I always give patients the options with some information, and then let them decide what they want to do . . . most women are very well versed in HRT nowadays. What they don't understand is when to have the oestrogen, and the actual mechanics of taking the tablets. They are not too clued up on the side-effects of the tablets. So, I always go through the side-effects with them, so they understand.

KNOWLEDGE

It is on the third dimension of the biomedical model that our data most clearly departs from the critical stereotype. None of these doctors appealed to 'pure' science over women's experience, indeed many of them seem troubled, even baffled, by the epidemiological debates they tried to keep track of. Each stressed individual difference and the need for detailed consultation with patients. But the tone of these accounts varied widely.

The statements about medical evidence range from absolutely confident to very diffident and anxious. Confidence could combine oddly with the understanding that there was no basis for it:

Well there is a lot of controversy. There is still controversy expressed in the medical journals I read, however, I feel that the consensus is that hormone replacement therapy, properly prescribed and properly adhered to, is safe and effective and I personally don't have any doubt about its use.

None of the doctors mentioned personal experience; three, all from the working-class area, cited professionals as sources of information, only one the literature. One general practitioner said it was hard to put the ideas in his own words, 'I suppose I've attended too many seminars.' 'You're a groupie?' I asked, referring to the apparently unending roadshow of menopause information sessions. He answered sharply:

> No, I'm not a groupie. I'm actually quite sick of it. I think it is overdone. I think other areas are lacking attention. I think menopause is getting too much attention. I think the push for hormone replacement is too strong compared to the push for other things.

Some doctors showed a clear resistance to the task of evaluating the 'scientific' evidence. They either said they were not capable of doing this, or asserted that it wasn't their job. However, most doctors had a current 'position' on the safety of HRT, and very few told us it is entirely safe. However, the language they used is interesting: 'pretty well safe', 'quite safe'. A female doctor of Italian origin gave a cheerful verdict: 'I think that it is probably quite safe; otherwise we wouldn't be using it.'

Only five mentioned the risks of HRT. Only one discussed the cost of treatment. It was clear that some doctors felt they were unable to access recent scientific evidence or even sometimes the evidence of the patient. The language of one male doctor certainly suggested the patient was more a laboratory than a person:

> A few would come in with those symptoms, and then we would talk about whether it was menopausal. I think if they are late forties early fifties, there is always the possibility that those symptoms may be helped with hormones. But, we would need to have a few more symptoms . . . I'd like to have some flushes and some dryness and sexual problems with that . . . I'd like to have it, but sometimes, you don't. You've got to work out if you are going to go into pharmaceutical, whether you are going into anti-depressants or oestrogens.

POWER

The fourth and final cluster of ideas in the biomedical stereotype is the hardest to examine. Power, control and authority are extremely difficult to locate in data, and this is particularly true of data about clinical settings. The terminology of medical prescription and supervision reeks of authority, and many of the doctors we talked to indicated by their choice of words that they anticipated unquestioned acceptance of their authority. 'I order HRT' said one male. Others used phrases that indicate patriarchal assumptions back their conviction of medical authority.

There is, however, no interview that fits the 'biomedical' stereotype of patriarchal power. Almost all of the doctors remark, sometimes with interest, sometimes with annoyance, on women's ability to self-diagnose and obtain information from other sources. As Kaufert (1982) comments, this can be a problem:

> From the medical perspective, it is essential that a woman's confidence in her own ability to interpret her experience be undermined. She must be convinced that only a physician can correctly diagnose whether she is menopausal. (p. 151)

Most doctors we interviewed said they encouraged women to interpret symptoms and make decisions. Some explicitly said they avoid the responsibility of deciding for them:

> I find this difficult really because if you push women into hormone replacement therapy and they then get problems, the doctor then feels almost responsible for their problems. So I give the woman all the information and let her make the choice. If she asks for my advice, what I would do if I was in her situation, well then I would happily give the advice. But I don't like pushing them into taking it in case they run into problems of abnormal bleeding or some trouble that requires them to have [an] investigation such as a curette. Now the worst situation I can find myself in is being over emphatic that you ought to take the hormones and then she reluctantly, on my advice, goes out and takes these oestrogens and perhaps we run into a bit more bleeding than we thought we might and then I'm placed in the situation of recommending that she goes out and has a curette.

On the other hand, much of the language is about the doctor's ability to guide that decision, and there is a fine line between guidance and dogmatism. A woman general practitioner says:

> I find that quite a lot of people are interested in hormone replacement treatment and knowing a little bit about that. So then I would touch on the options that are available . . . always specifying or giving them further information and literature to read . . . I say to them that if they decide on any medical treatment, hormone replacement treatment, there is something that we do need to discuss and that is not something, just because they are menopausal they get medication.

When do they get it, then? Her account suggests a quite difficult negotiation, in which she has the final say:

> It depends if they are symptomatic and if they are at risk of things, for example like osteoporosis, which then introduces preventative medicine. We talk about bone scans and things. But I know at the moment, it is very — hormone replacement treatment has been given a lot of press and I think it is very important to gauge how a woman feels about it. If I find that they are feeling okay or that they are not feeling so good but then [are] very reluctant to have hormone replacement and there is no risk to their health, then I certainly wouldn't push that.

In the mostly middle-class area, another female doctor remarked wryly that the patients in her practice included well-educated and informed women and 'lots and lots of doctors' wives': 'Some people would come with the idea that they are coming to get hormone replacement and they've done their reading and they have done their research and that's what they want.'

A male doctor's choice of words made his attitude clear: 'An awful lot of women have complete control of their medication, despite having been on it for long times, and they often give themselves a break.' Stories from women interviewed suggest that other women send hundreds of pills down the toilets of Victoria, but we talked to few who had done it themselves. Five told us they had thrown out pills after deciding they didn't understand or want hormone treatment which, as one put it, 'the doctor conned me into'. But there are also strong themes of women's resistance to what they see as unreasoning medical authority: turn from the interviews with doctors to the accounts from women and you find a different picture of medical dominance.

WHAT DID THE WOMEN SAY? NEGOTIATING AUTHORITY

Kaufert (1986) concluded ten years ago that despite the limitations of survey data, a study of Canadian women showed a wide range of behaviour by both women and physicians in response to menopause issues. Only a minority of women had treatment 'much as prescribed by the biomedical model, that is, one closely supervised by their physicians and involving the use of estrogen replacement therapy . . . In general, the experience of menopause was not a highly medicalized process and was one in which some women involved their physicians not at all.' (p. 16) She compared menopause with pregnancy: it is less visible, with some choice about whether or why it is hidden, and it is less associated with an agreed path of medical care. Importantly, she suggests, 'Just as women are not under the same pressure to seek medical care when they are menopausal as when they are pregnant, physicians also have more freedom . . . physicians are not yet under pressure — whether legally or by their colleagues — to keep estrogen levels at some pre-defined level. A physician can be sued for not doing a Caesarian section; he cannot be sued for failing to prescribe hormones.'

Some of the doctors we talked to disagreed, and one gave this as a strong reason for not arguing against hormone treatment. However, the women we talked to never raised this sort of threat. Rather, their accounts suggest that the freedom to avoid or subvert the advice of their general practitioners is both a problem and a challenge for them. Unrestrained by the survey format, the women we interviewed sometimes gave detailed accounts of their negotiations with medical authority. We turn now from the doctors' voices, and back to the women's.

It is clear from these accounts that very many women thought their doctors were unwilling or unable to understand the

of menopause and the HRT decision for them. One
ᴅ us her doctor had talked about HRT, but for her it
ₓpensive. She couldn't afford the cost of the tablets, and
as ₛ₊ as already taking four different types of tablets for her
health she didn't want to take any more. She also felt that it may
be a risk for her. Another had been put on Premarin for stress,
and went back when symptoms returned. 'He gave me a different
tablet. It was a German one. But I never took it, and haven't taken
it since.' Another put it graphically, 'I wasn't too sure he was
totally sympathetic. I felt his attitude was inclined to be a bit "give
her some hormones and she'll piss off."'

It was also clear that many of the women we talked to had
developed, in conversation with other women, a (newly?) dis-
respectful attitude to medical authority. Male general practitioners
in particular were regarded as fallible, and the language women
used to tell their stories was often vivid, relating strong messages
that general practitioners talk down to women and misread their
body changes:

> My sister is on the patch . . . She said that before she went to the
> clinic, she was getting a lot of bladder infections, and she told the
> doctor in there. When she went to her own doctor, he used to put her
> on antibiotics and say, 'Off you go.' Of course, when she told the
> [women's clinic] doctor, they said, 'No, that doesn't seem right.' They
> said, 'I think we'll put you on the patch.' She's been on that now for
> three months, and she feels wonderful. She hasn't had any bladder
> infection . . . The doctor was feeding her antibiotics, and since she's
> been on the patch, she hasn't had one . . . She believed in her doctor,
> so she took them. But, she's not all that keen on taking antibiotics . . .
> She took them because she wanted to get rid of her bladder infection.
> But, now, she is of the same opinion that I am, that you really don't
> go to your local GP. You go to specialised women's clinics.

The processes of resistance are subtle. Just the choice of words
here contains rebellious messages: the doctor had doubtless not
said, 'Off you go', and was not 'feeding' the antibiotics to her as
to a baby. We were struck by the language of rebellion against a
collective authoritative 'they', especially in the accounts from less-
educated women:

Oh they just say, 'Oh well, you know, take these and try these and see how you go', and when you go back and say, 'Well no, no, this doesn't work', the first [hormone treatment] that I was on, the male one, was dreadful. I was putting on 7 pound, fluid and I was just oh agro. So I went back and said 'NO!', you know, 'I am telling you'. He said, 'How do you know it's that?' and I said 'Because I am telling you it is when I take this ten day bloody male pill'. But you know, 'You are stupid, oh that can't happen' . . . So in the end you insist, 'I want to try something else.' Then they will give you something else. You are very lucky if you find a doctor that understands it and is willing to experiment with you.

Like the processes of transition work discussed in chapter 7, these processes of negotiation are clearly facilitated by resources, but not determined by them. Better-off women and women with education were more likely to have the confidence to debate or dodge doctors' instructions and question or challenge advice, to 'shop around' for other views, or make up their own minds, and more likely to have access to friends and literature they regarded as adequate alternative sources of information. They also seemed, not surprisingly, less likely to change on impulse, more likely to conduct what looked like research, using their networks and weighing views. But even these women showed how complex the processes could be and how many contributing decisions were made on impulse.

Sue's story has been told in part in chapter 7. She did not see herself as 'taking charge', but had remade her life in her late forties, both in terms of daily work and family pressures, and in terms of values. In the middle of this process she went through the HRT decision, and her detailed account gives a vivid picture of the complex factors involved. A medical friendship network and tertiary education makes it easy, almost too easy, to get information outside the patient role, and the words she uses indicate her uncertainty about its status ('I gather', 'the clincher that got me in', 'that clicked for me'). A sense of propriety about appointments and referrals, and her past casual attitude to medical advice, make it difficult to locate the advisers she now wants. Decisions made on impulse completely alter the framework of her health care. The result is that at the time of our interview she still is not sure she wants hormone treatment and may defy the medical advisers she has finally found:

> I thought, 'I don't need to muck around with HRT', so I didn't go down that path and before I knew what had happened my periods were back . . . Well I gather that is the scene anyway so it tends to come and go a bit and I just settled back to the way it had always been until a couple of months ago . . . I started experiencing some hot flushes again and I was at a party and I met a psychologist who actually works in the area of menopause, who I'd been at university with and we got to talking . . . and I told her that I wasn't going for HRT and she told me I was mad and she gave me a bit of a talking to and it finished up with . . . the clincher that got me in which was that we weren't meant to live into old age and so it is not unnatural tampering with the body, we are doing that by staying alive — and that clicked for me and I thought she is right, I should do it, particularly given the problems that my mother had with osteo-arthritis.
>
> So then the dilemma who to go and see, now you really get to the medical stuff. I thought about it for a few days and then I thought I would get an appointment with [a high-profile woman doctor] and then I would go and see my GP and ask him for a referral . . . And I was told the first appointment was in October . . . So I thought there was no point in going chasing after one of these big names . . . Well I will certainly not go back to my old gynae who every time I went to I felt I would never go back . . . I kept going mainly because I have never really had any problems or at least nothing I ever saw as problems . . . At one stage I discussed with my GP finding someone else in fact telling him I would like to see a woman and he [said], 'I don't understand this thing about women wanting to see women, a doctor is either competent or not competent. I know some incompetent women.' And he is not wrong, at one stage I tried to take one of my daughters to a local woman GP around the corner who proved to be a great disappointment to me — one of the worst consultations I have ever experienced. But I accepted his argument and I thought, 'Why start on another man, I might as well stay with the devil I know, who is remarkably understanding about women's problems I think.' And he is elderly now too which probably makes matters worse, it is the sort of, 'There, there, dear', pat on the head sort of stuff.

WHAT *DID* THE DOCTOR SAY? 193

Her attempt to find alternative advice thwarted, the next stage of the story interestingly contains belittling language: 'I went around' to the general practitioner, and 'trotted off home':

> So I went around to see my GP and . . . I discussed with him where I was at, which I hadn't had an occasion to do, and told him that I had decided against HRT but I was now changing my mind. And he said, 'Well I am changing my mind about HRT. I have been against it, I thought it was a licence for the drug companies to print money.' And I mean he is that sort of guy, he is very very concerned about it on a philosophical basis, about where medicine is going [,] particularly in the drugs area. And he said, 'I have now decided that old age is not a natural stage and so you have to help it along.' And I said, 'It is interesting that you say that Jim, because that is what has brought me here!' So we then had a debate about who invented that idea and he had never heard it before, and he just thought it up. And so having intended to get him to refer me on, he had obviously thought about it and he thought about those rates and he tried a few different things out and he seemed to know what he was doing and so I accepted his prescription and trotted off home with it.

The body behaved differently than expected; Sue did some self-diagnosing and acted against his advice:

> The only problem was . . . some abdominal discomfort so I went back to him and said, 'Do you think the dose is wrong?' And he said, 'Look I think at this stage . . . perhaps rather than changing the dose or stopping now just keep going and see what happens.' And so over the next few days I started to experience these pre-period dragging feelings and then we went away for the weekend for a friend's fiftieth birthday and . . . I had three days or something of this pain and I thought maybe these things are attacking my stomach. And I read the leaflet in the packet and saw that oestrogen could upset the system and so I thought I would just stop taking them. I mean I considered stopping under medical supervision. I thought no I don't want to take another one. Half the people there were doctors and I considered talking to one of them and then I thought, no, I just don't like mixing business and friendship. I thought just lay off them and see what happen[s], and things didn't improve.

In the last act of this small drama her account is more of 'agreements' with her advisers than instructions and, despite feeling uncomfortable, she finds a way to ask the general practitioner's advice about a change to a new adviser, heard of from women's conversations 'around the traps'. The woman doctor offers information in a way Sue finds 'reassuring':

> When I went to see my GP in fact what we agreed was that I would keep going but I said to him, 'Look I gather there is a GP in [a distant suburb] who is very interested in menopause who seems to have a lot of experience with it. How would it be if I went and discussed it with her?' I felt a bit uncomfortable talking to my doctor who has also become a family friend in that light, but needless to say he said, 'I think that is a good idea.' Last year when I was talking to these older friends, one of them gave me her name along with [high-profile woman doctor] and said, 'Look these are two people whose names are around the traps who some of my friends are seeing or hearing speak' ... So in fact by the time I went to see her, which had been intended just to see what sort of drug regimen I should be on, it turned into a full-blown investigation of what all these abdominal pains were, and for me it was a very interesting experience for the first time ever interacting with a doctor who asked lots of questions, [took] the full medical history, was interested in every facet of life and took a holistic approach and had an understanding of HRT. And she explained in great detail, she drew graphs and explained dose levels and aims and objectives of therapy and what sort of regimens would achieve different patterns as far as having periods and not having periods or having three-monthly periods or whatever was the concern. And I, it was really one of the most reassuring consultations I have ever had with a doctor, reassuring in the sense that I felt that she knew what she was doing and also was capable of communicating it ...

A happy ending? Not so simple. The HRT decision has still not been made. At the time of the interview she had changed doctors but retained the sort of partial control so many women had, to guide the decisions that her bodily changes demanded (a strange sort of control this, rather as an inexperienced canoeist, swept downriver, is able to guide the canoe through rapids, but always downstream):

> As time has gone on I have seen her a few times because she was keeping a close watch on these abdominal cramps, which suddenly disappeared last Saturday and haven't reappeared, so what they were we don't know, whether they were related to the oestrogen or not I

don't know. But in fact she has given me a prescription for the oestrogen patch, she feels I shouldn't take it orally . . . So actually I have not gone back on to it, because once again I am feeling better. Well actually what has happened is I have stopped taking it! . . . I haven't had a period, I haven't had any hot flushes and so I said to her on Monday after all this pain business had stopped, 'Look, I would really like to just settle back. I am actually feeling good for the first time since I started on the HRT, what if I leave it a few weeks? I will start taking it when I feel like it.' And then I will go back and see her after I have been on it for a month. So no I am not on it at the moment.

I asked if the new doctor recommended staying on HRT, and Sue said as though the answer was obvious, 'Oh permanently, forever.'

THE BIOMEDICAL BACKDROP

How to interpret this data? The only clear conclusion is that there is no single biomedical model behind the doctors' interpretation of their role, and that the women have no single perception of doctors' authority. But while some of the critiques of the biomedical perspective have appeared to claim it dominates *all* practice, this is not how dominant ideologies usually work. Variety of practice does not mean that medical practice is free of the strands of ideology identified in the critique. The biomedical model can be seen as a backdrop to the daily pressures of practice for the doctors, and dilemmas and decisions for the women.

Nor do expressions of good intent mean they are reflected in practice. It is easy to find, from most (though indeed not all) of the doctors, statements of their holistic approach and their refusal (for one of many very different reasons) to make decisions for women. But it is not possible to guess how these intentions translate in practice.

By emphasising variety of interpretations, and the ubiquity of expressions of good intentions, it would then be easy to dismiss the critique of medical authority as irrelevant. Looked at one way, through their own words, these are indeed doctors whose exercise of power is appropriate to their superior knowledge, and whose directive behaviour is required for the patient's good, but who are also able to see the 'whole' patient when appropriate. Such a pragmatic model of medical interaction is proposed by Maseide (1991) and has been used in a short thesis examining these same twenty interviews to conclude that:

> We have a group of doctors who are more than aware of their social responsibilities . . . sensitive to the needs of their patients and attempt to be as responsive as possible. At the same time they are more than aware that there are times in general practice when, if only for reasons of medical ethics and responsibility, they become directive with some of their patients. (Simon 1994, p. 41)

This generous verdict hardly fits some of the material quoted above, and overlooks considerable variety in the data. Many of the doctors were confused about treatments and expressed concern that they did not know enough. Looked at less generously, their confidence in their skills of clinical interaction or the pressure of time seem in some cases to allow dismissal of women's experiences and glossing of their own ignorance. Our data strongly supports Kaufert's warning, 'It is easy to fall into the trap of ascribing an inappropriate form of reality to the biomedical model' (1986, p. 17), but this is not to deny the background relevance of this model. The stories in previous chapters tell of practically every sort of interaction between woman and doctor, and analysis of the words they use suggests a very wide range of understandings of the doctor–patient relationship. In each of the areas where we interviewed, there were some women like Jess who saw their doctors as dogmatic and unprepared to discuss; and there were some women who said their doctors were aware and sensitive. At the other extreme from the stereotype of dictator doctor, a persistent theme was women's reporting doctors' refusals to dictate decisions, especially about HRT. Some appreciated this, but others were puzzled, worried or angry, and did not wish for the control being offered them.

Looked at another way, these data are inadequate to the task of assessing the critique of the 'biomedical perspective'. It is easy to find quotations that support a blanket clearance of the doctors from the 'biomedical' charge. However, although we would hardly expect the doctors to utter obviously patriarchal statements hostile to women's health in the present context, it is startlingly easy to find in their accounts assumptions about medical care and menopause, knowledge and power, that are part of the biomedical stereotype. While Maseide's model usefully directs us to the pragmatic demands of medical practice, it should not divert us from the pervasiveness of those ideas of the biomedical model and the task of understanding how women receive and respond to them, and the effects they have on health practice.

Our data indicate the increasing vulnerability of general practitioners' authority, and their insecurity about not knowing all the facts (two told us they were anxious about HRT but that the patients would go elsewhere if they expressed uncertainty). We were shown a range of ways in which women dodged or dealt with medical authority, by shopping for doctors or shifting to 'natural' therapy. We gained a picture of doctors' discomfort with, even hostility to, women's knowledge, gleaned from friends or reading, lectures and information nights, and of difficulties they met in reasserting their proper place as gatekeepers to knowledge when knowledge is seen as debatable and questionable. And behind all this was a picture of a problem area of practice, of the messiness of menopause, publicly debated, with uncertain epidemiology, symptoms that persist but are not life threatening and involving a decision, an apparent choice. Four doctors expressed some degree of irritation about the 'industry' of writing and information on menopause.

A male doctor summarised, 'It is easier to put her on HRT; then she walks out the door and, in a way, you have solved the problem.' But he was not suggesting that this is what he did. The wider context was also provided:

> She still might have problems even though she is on the therapy and even though you are controlling her symptoms. There might be other things as well . . . You still have to keep that in the back of your mind, that she is not going to walk out feeling 'Oh, wow, I'm great now!' and things are good, because often they are not.

It could be argued that many doctors quoted trivialise women's problems and knowledge, but more sound extremely anxious not to be seen as doing so. A stronger theme is the doctors' own uncertainty and lack of information, in situations where their patients have access to knowledge of varying origin and perceived reliability. We were surprised by the very common comments about women following other women, a 'bandwagon' effect, in going onto HRT. In very brief interviews it is hard to assess these. They might indicate displeasure at women's discovering sources of information outside the doctor's control. These comments, however, indicate much more complicated processes by which patients negotiate their medical knowledge with doctors. Some of the questions raised cannot be answered without different data, allowing detailed interpretation of doctor behaviour in a range of circumstances, studying how it changes in response to the need for authority and direction, and how those needs are assessed by both patient and doctor, and the behaviours interpreted by both.

The 'biomedical perspective' seems then to be a political label for a much less formidable, much more fluid, changing and challenged set of ideas that hang as a largely unnoticed backdrop to doctor–patient relations. Ideology is of course most effective when neither seen nor resisted. To say there is an ideological backdrop to clinical practice is not to say individual doctors are uncaring or that women are dupes of medical myths and dictator doctors. Women's accounts, in this and previous chapters, showed their differing degrees of agency in managing clinical interactions. They used a range of strategies to deal with authoritative knowledge, including accepting it and reinterpreting it as specifically acceptable to their situation, appearing to accept and then undermining it, supplementing, arguing and confronting it. The backdrop for some was awareness of doctors' uncertainty and confusion. For other women, whose experiences of help-seeking had been painful and problematic, the backdrop was a rigid relationship of authority and lack of communication. Those backdrops changed for some women with experience, constantly rewoven from different combinations of the threads of care, relationships, knowledge, power.

10
ANOTHER SORT OF CARE? COMMUNITY LEVEL ADVICE

Lyn Richards

The previous chapter established that doctors spoke with (and women heard) many adviser-voices on midlife, few from the stereotypical biomedical perspective. While some doctors expressed views close to the stereotype, and some women told stories suggestive of it, there is no evidence that women in this study uniformly, or even, to our surprise, commonly, suffered from medical advice hostile to women's special social contexts and producing narrowly medical solutions. To make that assumption would be to risk ignoring varieties of experience and context, which may be crucial to understanding and improving women's health as well as varieties of concern, curiosity and uncertainty by doctors, which certainly need to be noted and addressed.

Just this assumption about medical advice, however, pervades arguments for a different level of health care at 'grass roots' or 'community level', a level often seen as special to women's health issues. The women's health movement has actively promoted this level as 'a solution to problems which women have experienced in mainstream medical model health services'. (Hunt 1991, p. 2)

Variously portrayed as more 'holistic', less limited by the biomedical perspective and more accessible to women, this level of advice is located in some formal settings (community health centres, citizen's advice bureaux [CABs]) and many informal or irregular ones (community house meetings, women's groups, church groups, occasional help sessions or information nights). At the community level, health-care advice is offered by nurses in many different employment settings, and by administrators and untrained or trained helpers. This chapter looks first at the models of community level care. How is this sort of care different? Then it focuses on our data from advisers at that level. Do women go there for help and, if they do, what help are they offered?

THE CLAIMS FOR COMMUNITY CARE

There is now a substantial literature asserting that community level care can and/or must offer a different style, content and process of health care from that offered by medical clinics and general practitioners. In Australia, nurses have been urged since the 1970s to see their role as promoting wellness and health, rather than just caring for the ill (Baum, Fry & Lennie 1992). This has been presented as a 'paragdigm shift' whereby nurses in particular replace a 'curative model' with a 'holistic' one. The reach of these models is dramatic, and their attainment clearly would demand massive rethinking and resource reallocation:

> In health care, it would consist of restoring and maintaining the dynamic balance of individuals, families and other social/community groups. It would also mean people taking care of their own health individually, as a society, and with the help of therapists, that is, by Greek definition, 'comrades in a common struggle'. This kind of health care cannot just be 'provided' or 'delivered', it has to be practised. (do Rozario 1994, p. 6)

By the 1990s, an enquiry on community nursing education could assert this new role with confidence:

> The essence of the CHN [community health nurse] role is one which encapsulates the philosophy of community health. It is characterised by a holistic approach towards health care, with a concern for the community's and the individual's physical, environmental, emotional,

social, psychological and economic health. (Post-registration (Nursing) Education Advisory Committee 1991, p. 33)

But practice seemed to lag behind. The enquiry found a high proportion of managers of community health-care centres showed 'adherence to a medical model (that is a concentration on illness rather than wellness) was enforced, with very little comprehension of the wide range of areas of work appropriate to a CHN' (p. 34). Nurses too were confused. Only some could 'clearly articulate the essence of their role' (p. 36) and few had chosen it for the preferred reasons of philosophy of community health and the focus on prevention, or disillusionment with 'the limitations and emphasis of the medical model' (p. 22).

This may be because the ideal is unclear: statements of community health roles (rather like statements of the biomedical perspective), prove very inconsistent. The common word in all these presentations appears to be 'holistic', but that seems to mean many things to writers and practitioners (each carrying implied contrast with medical consultation). It can refer to approaches encompassing social and environmental factors beyond the 'narrowly' medical; thus a 'holistic approach' to menopause services meant approaching 'whole persons' rather than body parts, and including social transitions and contexts in consideration. Or it can refer to ongoing communication and consultation. Thus one program was described as 'holistic, and has an individualised approach', because the team assumed 'many factors were involved in promoting health and preventing disease for the menopausal women' and aimed at addressing 'the need for women to be provided individual, unhurried assessment. It was believed this assisted in promoting dignity and self worth of the woman.' (Ashcroft & O'Brien 1992, pp. 27–8)

The four themes identified in the previous chapter as parts of the model of the biomedical perspective reappear here as shown in Figure 10.1. But interestingly the community health model is not merely a flip side of the biomedical. The ideal of community health is no mere rejection of the biomedical, but has its own positive themes. Where medical care is claimed to emphasise illness treated with drugs, the ideal of community level care is well-

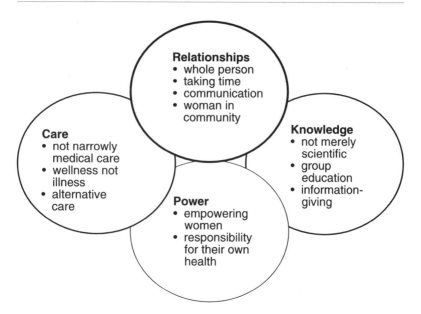

Figure 10.1 Themes in the ideal model of 'community-level health care'. (Compare Figure 9.1, p. 176.)

ness and care in context. Where the doctor–patient relationship is seen as impersonal, community health offers holistic care, the carer constructing ongoing relationships with the 'whole person'; and where scientific knowledge is seen as cut-and-dried, self-knowledge, 'alternative' medicine and shared knowledge is emphasised. Where doctors' power is rejected, the new theme is empowerment of women, and 'responsibility for own health'.

There is an obvious affinity between values regarding community nursing roles and values in the women's health movement (Broom 1991). On the basis of interviews in nine countries, Hunt (1991) concluded that the women's health movement was shaped by three dominant ideologies, feminism, empowerment ('the dimensions of which include: knowledge; skills; social action; new forms of organisation; resources and access to resources'), and 'the social model of health which links health issues to broader social structures' (p. 2).

Exploring the Community Level

Our data from women just didn't fit these ideological statements. Despite the strong messages about preferable health care for women, and evidence that community care was focusing on menopause, we did not find one woman in the first year of our project who talked about obtaining advice from these sources. The experience of menopause in almost all women's accounts was of individual decisions or lack thereof, informed by medical knowledge conveyed almost entirely by general practitioners.

This data tended to confirm the impression given in much of the literature that women experience menopause in isolation from other women's experiences and learn about it mainly through consultation with doctors. Women we spoke to in groups or individually sought advice from doctors or acquired it, sometimes without seeking, from friends, or did without it. Not one had taken midlife or menopause related issues to community level advisers or nurses, or even acquired knowledge from such sources without seeking it. None of them hinted at relevance of health professionals other than doctors or 'alternative' practitioners (naturopaths, chiropractors, homoeopaths). Nurses simply did not appear as advisers: no woman mentioned getting health advice from a nurse. In the survey, we asked women to circle on a list of health professionals all those they go to for health advice. The least often nominated was nurse, circled by only 14 women (or 1.3% of the sample), 8 of these in age groups under 35.

The apparent irrelevance of community health could be explained in many ways. Our sampling of women was very skewed to the middle class; were community advisers relevant in less well-off areas? Did women not know they could get advice at the community level? Was it not available on this topic? Did they not want it?

We went looking for it. In the second half of 1991, we set out to map advice at community level by telephone interviews with advisers, by attending the menopause information events we learned of, and by talking to the women who went to them.

Working from lists of community services, a woman interviewer telephoned every community health centre and citizen's advice bureau in the Melbourne metropolitan area, asking for the person who handled requests for advice on menopause.

The results were startling both in terms of the quality of the data and its content. The project produced 83 interviews (45 with nurses in community health centres, 13 with nurses in hospitals, 11 with advisers in CABs, 10 with community house representatives, 3 at information centres and 1 in a women's health cooperative). The brief transcripts gave vivid pictures of areas of confidence, uncertainty, goals and frustrations. We also attempted to attend or learn about social groups or information sessions mentioned in phone interviews or advertised in local papers. Fifteen single information nights and meetings were observed and a team member took part in one series of eight information sessions as a participant observer. We built up a collection of pamphlets distributed to women at sites contacted.

Far from presenting a single community-level process, these interviews indicated virtually every possible approach, from complete ignoring of the issues we asked about through to total focus on them, from any of an equally wide range of perspectives. More centres addressed questions about menopause than not. In a few centres (mainly those focusing on the needs of very young communities) a nurse — or CAB adviser — saw it as odd or surprising that we should ask about advice on menopause. Most, however, saw it as central, and reported that women did come for information, and were given it:

> Women usually present if they are in the age group or if they have unpleasant symptoms. They walk in seeking information. The nurse gives them information the first time, the woman reads it. This satisfies the immediate request. Then they may return saying, 'I've tried these it hasn't worked what else can I do?' Or they may say, 'I've seen HRT talked about or written about in the media, what about that?' After a discussion I usually refer [them] to a local GP.

About half saw the topic as having unusual significance among women's health issues, either because of the demographic pattern of the local community or because it was a matter of current debate, a preferred issue for workshops discussing health. Often a professional, always a woman, almost always a community health nurse, had taken initiative in setting up women's groups or information meetings on menopause. These women all stressed the goals of 'validating' women's experiences, offering alternatives to, or a wider perspective than, medical views.

A DIFFERENT SORT OF HEALTH CARE?

Data dissolves stereotypes! The previous chapter showed that women visiting general practitioners rarely had an experience that fitted any of the four idea-sets in the narrowly medical stereotype. More often, they were directed to make up their own minds about HRT, or dissuaded from it. Most doctors claimed to take a wide range of factors into account in advising women, and almost all reported some concerns about HRT.

This chapter draws on a different body of data — our interviews, mostly by phone, with community health advisers. Quotations are, unless otherwise indicated, from notes taken by the interviewer during these interviews. Each of the four themes in the community health model will be explored in turn through this data.

CARE — REJECTING THE MEDICAL?

We found eight advisers, all women and all nurses, whose practice apparently followed the holistic community-health model perfectly. But other advisers made it clear that women visiting a community centre might get treatment that is nearer the biomedical stereotype, including immediate referral to doctors and apparently common advocacy of hormone prescription. Indeed we found it increasingly difficult to distinguish two different types of health care.

One health clinic 'with a community focus' held a weekly menopause session. The receptionist said the clinic was 'run on the medical model', a patient would see one of the female doctors, who had 'a community focus to their work'. This meant they 'do not just focus on disease and treating the disease, but work in a model which focuses on other areas of the person's life, the doctor is more likely to incorporate counselling and information-giving in this style of practice'. The women who attend the menopause clinic are given time to discuss their concerns. She described it as a 'marvellous area' in which to work. 'The women come dragging themselves in and go out bouncing.' Many but not all would be prescribed HRT.

Even in our brief telephone interviews, health advisers varied so widely in their attitudes that it was impossible to find any ideas common to all. But as with the doctors' accounts, themes recurred in a way that showed the backdrop influence of the four sets of ideas pictured in Figure 10.1: ideas of care, of relationships, of knowledge, and of power. The following sections deal with each of these in turn.

The most dramatic difference between the ideal and reality of the community-health model is in the attitudes to medical care. The advisers we talked with in telephone interviews usually saw their work as collaborative with doctors. Only four compared what they did to a medical model (interviewers' notes are quoted here and below):

> She felt many older women who had been socialised into the medical model were 'sucked into HRT'. She had 'come across women who had been on HRT for fifteen or twenty years' and their medication had not been reviewed, these were older women 65 to 70 years. They had 'medicos sitting on a pedestal'.

On the other hand several nurses indicated that they saw general practitioners as behind, or less informed than, or less perceptive than, nurses in understanding of menopause:

> She said that there were still many GPs who did not have very much knowledge of the menopause, that very often the attitudes were that the symptoms were not menopause, because the women were either too young, too old. Put the women on tranquillisers, or the women should just put up with the symptoms and accept [them].

If the advisers accurately described the care they offered, in some areas women are more likely to get advice that is 'just medical' at the community level than from their local doctor. In others, the community level adviser acts simply as a conduit to general practitioner consultation. And where biomedical responses are given, they are more often unquestioned in these accounts than in the interviews with doctors.

Over half of the advisers we talked to referred women to general practitioners, and none of these expressed any concern about medical advice. There were, however, many ways of referring. Some did so without questioning the authority of the doctor or knowing anything about the advice given. Others made it their business to get information on local general practitioners, in four cases to find women doctors. Some nurses saw their tasks as including a watchdog role in monitoring medical advice:

> The centre is working within the dual strategy framework: working with professionals to change attitudes to women; influencing GPs, nurses, both in the community and in hospital. If they hear of a service provider who has treated a woman in a paternalistic manner, the centre contacts that person to try to change the attitude.

Two said they referred in the context of informing the women about how to communicate with doctors, or medical options:

> I asked her if she received referrals from the local GPs. She said, 'No, not yet, we send the women back to the GPs.' This happened when the women had concerns but didn't know how to ask the right questions of their doctors. It took a while to get the group working.

Overall, statements of faith in medical solutions and assertion of unquestioned medical authority are as easy to find in this body of data as in doctors' or women's accounts of what doctors said. However, alongside this is an insistence on seeing menopause in context. It is striking that HRT occurs as a much more contentious issue in these interviews than in the doctors'.

The significance of the HRT issue at community level rapidly became evident. In some of the telephone interviews it was the only issue raised by the adviser, or other issues were couched in that context. The affirmation of women's experience and understanding of 'total context' did not stop community level advisers from recommending HRT. However all who did so insisted it should be one thing of many that women considered. One nurse described it as 'a lifesaver' but said she always suggested women learn about it for themselves. Another commented:

> The women are on it just because their doctor says they should go on it. The women phone querying its use. She felt that HRT has its place. However she felt that it should not be pushed upon the women, the women need to know about HRT. She said she gave the women information pamphlets, books.

Several advisers said they aimed to encourage women to think for themselves about the advice they hear from doctors:

> Her approach was to suggest to the women that they go to the doctor for diagnosis, the diagnosis gives them control, then she encouraged the women to choose what treatment they wanted. She felt that it was interesting why certain people choose different treatments.

But the nurse took no agency in the choice. Most sent the woman to the doctor first, then encouraged thinking about the advice. In a taped interview, a nurse gave a detailed account:

> I don't present it as the first bit of information. The women may ask, the doctor put me on these tablets, what are they? In this situation I find out what they are and what they have been told and take it from there, I try not to antagonise the relationship with [the] Medico. I suggest if they want more info that there is a clinic at the Women's because it is more specialised, and let the women know they can go [there] for clinical services. I suggest the Women's because it's near and they can walk. I have seen a woman who was going to stop her HRT, she sees her GP regularly and she had been given unopposed oestrogen.

Very few advisers expressed an unequivocal attitude to hormone treatment, but there were frequent comments that implied doctors 'pushed' HRT on women:

> G. suggested a better approach was to get the women to look at how they used to be compared with now. HRT was often looked upon as

the easy way out, instead of looking at the total. Women often felt that the loss of a partner's desires could be remedied with HRT. She had a question mark about the current push towards younger women starting HRT. She felt that there was an increased number of women informed about HRT. She felt that the women need[ed] adequate information. She had some concerns about cancer associated with HRT.

WELLNESS

In the literature on community-level health care, a strong theme is wellness rather than illness. Certainly the contextualising of menopause gave an opportunity for advisers to address this theme. But 'wellness' is markedly absent from these accounts. Context means a range of possible illnesses and fears, often startlingly negative. Even when 'total context' was sought, there was a strikingly narrow range of topics discussed in most of these groups. The agenda of information sessions almost always included a litany of physical deteriorations.

We asked all the community level advisers what they saw as symptoms of menopause. All cited physical signs, but most included psychological and/or social changes:

> She said: hot flushes, dry vagina, loss of concentration, confusion, feeling worthless, loss of self-esteem. Each of the groups was different. Aching joints, insomnia, irritability, looking old — feel[ing] life ends ... The concept is not clear about what to expect at menopause.

By the end of the project we had catalogued sixty-one symptoms of menopause, which as a team member remarked was enough to put you off it for life! Most were unambiguously unpleasant or unattractive, and it was this list of 'set things', as one nurse put it, that set the agenda for groups:

> A lot of women are not affected at all, some are affected a lot and some of the issues can also be experienced at other ages and stages of life. However there are set things when oestrogen does run down. There are the emotional areas. It's very complex. Physical symptoms, depression, bones brittle, hot flushes, increase in infections — UTI [urinary tract infection], incontinence, itchy skin, dry vagina, pain with intercourse, hair more brittle, skin wrinkles, more prone to insomnia.

In many statements, the 'total context' being 'normalised' was ageing. The nurses especially seemed to see their contribution as helping women to reject societal images of youth and beauty, and urging acceptance of ageing:

> She told of her experience recently with Jewish women where the topic was 'When does life begin?' There was an older group with women up to 80 years of age and the second group were younger, 45 to 55 years. The theme was interesting. The women talked about ages, stages, responsibility, their thought processes, the positive things about age. The younger group of women felt like the meat in the sandwich, waiting in fear. They were trying to be youthful, they were incredibly affected by the media, they were concerned about wrinkles and were not wanting to admit to age. Whereas the older women described it as the third stage of life, who cares, that's all behind us. The women were feeling complete and they had the benefits of life's experiences. The younger women were influenced by image and couldn't see age as enrich[ing]. [They wanted] to see themselves as pre-bride.

A final difference between these interviews and those with doctors was that the community level providers were sharply aware of the different issues for women from non-English speaking backgrounds.

> She felt that in respect to ageing that many had taken on attitudes of the Australians. She felt that the women's stories of menopause were much the same. The aim of the groups was to give the women an understanding of common symptoms such as change in periods, headaches, tiredness, depression, hot flushes and that the women in the groups talked of symptoms with which they were comfortable. J. said that women in groups do not mention sexual aspects as these would be seen as an embarrassment.

None of these themes occurred in the doctors' interviews.

'ALTERNATIVE' CARE

> There are lots of different things. Offer options, different choices. An eclectic model of services, explore women's needs. If flotation is the need or a dip in the sea we support the women with this need. There is certainly a place for alternative approaches. Whatever the woman wants we hope we can support the woman. There is a philosophical backing by the team for this approach.

Most advisers did not indicate such wide acceptance of all alternative health care. But in strong contrast to the interviews with doctors, the community-level interviews stress acceptance or at least tolerance of various forms of alternative medicine and that women should choose health care and take responsibility for their health. Naturopathy was the most common recommendation:

> Yes, D. said she would touch on naturopathy saying if it works for you that's terrific. D. felt that her role as an autonomous practitioner allowed her to give balanced information so that the women could make an informed choice.

The recommendation of 'alternatives' is always, however, within the context of the assumption of the validity of mainstream medicine. Advisers seemed to have a map of the medical system in which community health has a clear place. At the end of the holistic exploration, comes a referral:

> We look at women's experience of the medical system. The women's experience of menopause or life. We also run workshops on empowerment, so we run that as an adjunct to women's experiences, the myths and reality, and we provide information plus referral options.

Relationships

The second theme in the community care model is the one that most distinguishes the interviews with doctors from those with community level advisers. Where doctors largely ignored issues of their relationship with women patients, community level advisers were usually both concerned about and interested in relationships with women (and rarely called them patients). Three different strands appear: relationship with the 'whole person'; the significance of time; and the relevance of setting.

The whole person

The ideas about the 'whole person' and her context occurred in interviews with less than a quarter of the advisers at community level. But when they did occur they proved highly complex. The assertion that menopause should be seen in context was more common here than in our doctors' interviews, and it contained different themes. First, and most obvious, was that the experience of menopause was not merely one of biological change. One nurse said 'she felt that the main thing was to look at the total self. Treat symptoms as they come along, see menopause in the total context.' The total self and the total context is a big order, and nurses convinced that they should address these totalities commonly did so in very condensed agendas. This was especially so when advice was offered in groups, which usually met only once, or else covered many more health issues than just menopause.

A second sub-theme was more specifically about social transition. Six nurses commented that life is a continuum rather than 'segmented stages'. In one centre the nurse had organised groups which met weekly for five weeks. 'She included an overview of female physiology which she likes to keep brief (about five minutes). She included society's attitudes on women's issues and worked with the women in the group towards "normalisation of the menopause".'

'Total context' also had a third sub-theme. Some advisers hoped that by showing menopause as a 'normal' transition they could advance awareness of 'all the other things happening to women at that time'. Community talks were often described as focusing on menopause as 'a turning point in life'. A nurse who said 'she held a broad point of view' on HRT explained:

> People need to be comfortable with it. If there were problems, it can be useful. However not all women need to be prescribed treatment. She felt it was important to include nutrition and exercise [and] also to talk of the effects of the family maturing, and encouraged the women to see the time gained as time to develop creatively, if the women had a partner use the time to develop the partnership.

The language of 'whole woman' was not common in these interviews however. And when it occurred it was always associated with *giving* information rather than *relating* to the 'whole'. A nurse talked of her counselling role in terms of 'a focus on the whole health of the individual woman', exploring possible choices 'with an underlying emphasis on empowering the women'. She said she was interested in 'offering individual dignity to women'. She was one of very few nurses describing their work firmly in terms of the changing paradigms of community health. Another described the change to that paradigm — and the sense that it was not easily accepted:

> Currently she is working in consultation with local women to find out what is needed in health education and ... resources. This is part of the centre's move towards community development to see health issues in a broader context and health as focused on the whole being. It is a shift away from the identification of things such as osteoporosis, to more specific issues such as health issues for ageing, risks ... Menopause has not yet been raised. The women may view it as 'our lot and must go through it'.

TIME, TAKING AND GIVING IT

The patient in the waiting room is part of the backdrop to doctors' accounts. Listening and spending time is part of the discourse of community care:

> I asked if Julie sees women during menopause. She replied it was not the reason for coming, but that she sees a lot of women with menopause. 'We spend time talking with women about their health, in the process other issues are discussed. It's easy when talking about Pap smear procedure and they may talk about painful vaginas or we are just a friendly face to discuss these issues [with].'

Several nurses told of processes by which the topic came up, and emphasised that their role was to allow this to happen: 'K. replied that women did walk in and ask questions about menopause or they were seen for counselling and issues arose related to midlife. Some of the women presented with symptoms.' Listening is a word that occurs much more in these interviews than in those with doctors. One nurse said, 'we listen to women and speak with them, provide information and they can come in and use the literature — we have a lot of literature'. Another commented, 'I give women as much information as possible. I give them the opportunity to return if they need to chat further.'

SETTINGS AND COMMUNITY CONTEXTS

A related, and striking, difference from the doctors' interviews was that at least some of the community level advisers paid considerable attention to the settings of information sessions and consultations, and some did go 'into the community'. The difference is not surprising, as they are paid to do so. But their enjoyment of this role is obvious:

> She talked of one group with whom she worked at their workplace. Initially the group at this place of work had been very diverse with both English speaking and a large group of Greek women who were cleaners. She decided that because of the diversity of the group it would be much more satisfactory for all if she ran two separate groups. Once this had been achieved she had enjoyed the experience of communicating and getting to know the group despite having some difficulty with language.

The importance of being local was stressed by several advisers. Most encouraged local groups:

> She also said that she would like to see more support groups up and running in the local community. . . the local community houses were the place for these to be run. Apparently the distance to be travelled for the people in this area is the common complaint as to why they don't get help for a variety of problems. 'Women don't want to have to travel to the city from so far out.'

'Community' is one of the most commonly occurring words in this set of data, but it is hard to identify the community being accessed. The health-advice process seemed not to involve the local community beyond surveying demand for information on different topics. Community, in this context, rarely referred to local interaction or caring. None of the groups we attended were 'communal' in that sense. But while community figured little, proximity was often mentioned. Distance turned up several times as a theme, advisers commenting that they would refer women to a source of health advice nearby, assuming that distance is a deterrent. As one put it, she would not refer to a clinic further away because, 'You wouldn't want to travel.'

KNOWLEDGE

The third theme in the community care model offers strong contrasts with the medical model. Knowledge, especially knowledge acquired by group education and experience, is treated as a necessarily good thing in the community health literature, an assumption rarely discussed but clearly potent. The imperative that health education is properly done in groups was taken for granted by a large number of health advisers. Not one questioned the effectiveness of this form of caring or the comfortableness of women with group discussions on intimate topics. Several of the advisers we talked to had a cheerful routine of group process that they swung into whenever a group was scheduled:

> The nurse is about 45–50 years old. She is very interested in the area of menopause and has done a lot of work in the area as the 'specialist' nurse at the [community health centre]. I asked her about the format for the session tomorrow and she said that she usually opens each meeting with a 'brainstorming' session which differs according to the group. Tomorrow's group has about twelve women coming. She said that if the group appears to be largely women in their late thirties, she will start off with a discussion about PMS and use this as a vehicle to get to menopause. She also said that if the group appears to be in their late forties, she will dispense with this beginning and head straight into discussing and 'swapping' symptoms.

We had descriptions from eight centres of groups regularly run on women's health and/or menopause. There were two approaches used. One was a general 'whole context' approach, with emphasis on encouraging women to see their experiences broadly:

> We look at women's experience of the medical system. The women's experience of menopause or life. We also run workshops on empowerment, so we run that as an adjunct to women's experiences, the myths and reality, and we provide information plus referral options.

The second sort of workshop was concerned with women's bodies and their dysfunctions. The topics always seemed the same, an unhappy line-up of depressing subjects like brittle bones, stress incontinence and breast cancer. No woman was likely to suffer from all of these, but knowledge of all as threats might well be argued to depress and disrupt women and their efforts at redefinition of their selves at midlife. One centre:

> had run a half-day and full-day workshop on menopause. They also had a program about menopause one night per week for eight weeks. In the workshop a variety of professionals spoke: dietitians, and [a] physio talked on osteoporosis. The physio gives information on pelvic floor exercises and the link between lack of oestrogen and stress incontinence. The physio talks about exercise, walking and weight-bearing exercise. The nurse and social worker spoke on emotional issues.

Advertisements in local papers for menopause information sessions had the same foci — not a jolly picture, and not a likely set of topics to stimulate sharing of experience with strangers:

> The content of R's talk is to focus on midlife, areas of stress and the similarities between the symptoms of depression and menopause. Plus strategies for self-help, nutrition and exercise. [She also discusses] the need for increased calcium to guard against osteoporosis and [gives an] overview of HRT.

Knowledge is a recurrent theme in these interviews. And it is handled in a very similar way by a lot of those we talked to. There is a clear message in almost all of the telephone interviews that information is good, hence the more information a woman has the better. The record of one interview with a nurse compares sharply with the suggestion in at least some doctors' interviews that too much is either confusing or dangerous.

> When I asked her to explain her model of working with menopausal phase women she stated she worked from a base of allowing the women to make an informed decision. With individual women this is by talking about the pros and cons. She tries to give an overview of the subject including society's attitudes. In relationship to HRT she believed that it was certainly of benefit for women with symptoms

(approx. 1 in 10) and women at risk, however she emphasised that she did not see it as a 'quick fix' and the women were informed of this and the pros and cons.

There is also a strong suggestion that women's knowledge should supplement and extend beyond that given by a doctor. No community level advisers suggested this self-acquired knowledge should substitute for doctors' advice, but several were firm about the need to complement it:

> H's approach was to suggest to the women that they go to the doctor for diagnosis, the diagnosis gives them control, then she encouraged the women to choose what treatment they wanted. H. felt that it was interesting why certain people choose different treatments.

The handling of knowledge at this community level deserves more attention. There is a strong argument against regarding information as a commodity, an objective good, and consumers as 'input–output processors of information' (Dervin & Nilan 1986). In a different context (banking), Singh (1993) has argued this model of the informed consumer accessing and using information leads to dismal conclusions about consumer inadequacy. She suggests, following Dervin, focus on what users *call* information, and how they seek it.

> We ask users questions which start from our words, not theirs: What of the things we can do would you like us to do? What of the things we now offer do you use? The difficulty is that the data tell us nothing about humans and what is real to them. (Dervin 1992, p. 64)

Much of the debate on community health care is lit by the assumption that people (particularly women) are empowered by information provision. Many of those we talked to shared that assumption. It is less common for writers or advisers to ask what would be information, or what information would be empowering, or the conditions under which it would empower. Commonly there is an assumption that any information empowers, but little knowledge of what informs women. As menopause is such a popular topic for provision of information, there is an obvious danger that the women to whom this message is conveyed, if they hear the offer of information at the grass-roots level, can be overloaded rather than empowered by it. After her study of women's health movements in nine countries, Hunt observed, 'An overwhelming impression was that the world will soon collapse under the weight of literature about menopause'(1991, p. 6). She later observed that 'To be empowered, women need skills', nominating 'assertiveness, self-esteem and relaxation skills' (p. 7). Our data suggest that the skills needed also include the ability to find, to interpret and to see the relevance of information, and to ignore, bypass or store it away as well as to act on it.

Power

It is no new suggestion that power and knowledge are interlinked. In this case, the link seems to be between the advisers' insistence on *giving* knowledge and their refusal to claim authority, which in some cases seemed even evasion of power. There are two strong themes in this data.

Firstly, empowerment seemed to mean showing women they must take responsibility for their own health. This is one of the few themes in the model of ideal community-level health provision in Figure 10.1 that clearly recurs in the accounts from advisers.

Secondly, community level advisers were not merely unwilling to exert power: they often seemed afraid of doing so, unclear about the areas within which they had legitimate authority and anxious to defer to another (usually medical) source of authority.

'Responsible for your health'

What is it to be responsible for your health? It can have many meanings. The most common is the innocuous one that all possible options will be offered. Often this has a subtext: the adviser will not advise, but warns against taking (and in this case caricatures) medical advice:

> I then asked Margaret about HRT, she said she likes to talk of options and alternatives. It doesn't suit everybody. I give information and the

fors and againsts. There are lots of benefits from exercise, diet and increased calcium. HRT is very medicalised. Women are seen as a disease. I suggest to the women, 'Yes, it is good it does wonders for some women. It may not work for you.'

The ideal picture of the rational individual recipient being offered information which can be responsibly used fits our data badly in several respects, however.

As some of the quotations indicate, the information presented in literature or at information sessions was often technical and women who could not comfortably ask questions on intimate topics in a setting of strangers might not have understood it. (Each of us attending sessions had trouble with some of the medical vocabulary used!)

When the emphasis was on dispensing information as a commodity, at least some women had very negative responses to information sessions or printed materials, especially when they were unable to talk over what they learned. We noticed groups of women who already knew each other attending sessions: a friendship group from a high-income area, a church group in a semi-rural location, a business group that normally met for card games. Field notes from some group sessions comment on how much more comfortable women were if they arrived together.

The theme of being 'responsible for your health' is strongly repeated in this data. 'Women have a responsibility to learn about their body', says one nurse. The 'responsibility' theme often sounded as though an external force was imposing responsibility on the women. A nurse told groups of women, 'No one will ever be more concerned about your health than you. It's up to the individual to take responsibility for their well-being.' These two sentences provide an interesting insight into this theme: you are alone, you have to be competent.

What is it to 'take responsibility' for one's health? We can confidently take responsibility for a dog (train it and register it) or for a task (returning a book, arriving on time for a commitment), knowing that these are likely to remain within our control. Health is very different. Moreover, if the responsibility is placed on one person, they may be taking it *off* somebody else. (Relieving the physician of responsibility was, in this data, something women often did not want, and general practitioners did.) The language leans to the notion that someone once had the responsibility and now it has been given to the woman; therefore she must be responsible for and learn about her body. This shift personalises responsibility. What are the consequences of this? If you take responsibility you take the blame. You also take responsibility for the cost of being healthy because if you do not you will be a drain on the public purse.

Community level advisers clearly have considerable power. Though listening is a strong theme (fifteen women talked of this as their main role), it was always followed by advising. Even when the advice is referral, or instruction to take responsibility for your own heath, the adviser is affecting behaviour. When strong statements of 'grass-roots' care are made, the adviser exercises direction and purposiveness, determining the topics to be discussed, the way in which information will be given and the options presented, the opportunities offered and the pathways taken by the women 'clients': 'We intend setting up a program on health issues around ageing. We have found that if we call it menopause, the women don't come.' There is no mention in the community health model of the adviser's power: the efforts of community level advisers are aimed at empowering women, but the grammatical implications (*I* am empowering *you*) are not explored.

The apparently simple and wholesome themes of knowledge and empowerment turn out then to be much less dominant than the model suggests. The oft-derided term 'empowerment' actually turned up in our textual data only nine times. And then it proved less than simple. Once it was used by a woman doctor, concerned to avoid a narrowly medical stance:

> I think it really is about empowering people, that's I think our role. But there are some people that don't want to be empowered, and I have learnt that I have to be the doctor and they have to be the patient.

ONE STORY

In the late 1980s a women's health review stimulated activity in the semi-rural town where Rose was community health nurse. Five years on, she gives a vivid picture of a community level model at work, the sometimes extraordinary but often haphazard achievements of advisers working in this model and the problems they meet:

> Community health centres I think picked up on it because what women were saying in the consultation was that there wasn't enough information, there wasn't enough support for women in the midlife period . . . We organised a menopause seminar. It was our first big venture into doing an education program for women and we really weren't quite sure what was going to happen. We hired out the community hall and we did some publicity and advertised in the local rag. The day was pretty well structured around menopause and we had thirty-five women come along to that. That may not seem a lot of women but actually when we did our evaluation of the seminar and in the questionnaire, most of the women wanted to continue to gain more information in this area . . . Anyhow we had a meeting and we had some women attend that. There were some women that couldn't come for obvious reasons. It was decided that it would be an information-based group, not so much a support group. To me that sort of said that women were really hungry for information on the midlife period.

As several other organisers mentioned, success could be indicated only by attendance figures and evaluation comments. On the basis of these indicators, Rose's centre allocated resources to books, pamphlets and videos on midlife, and a women's health information group was formed, with the aim of a holistic approach to midlife needs. However, the thirty-five women seemed to have got what they wanted, and the midlife information effort caters now to a small group of stayers:

> It is actually going through a bit of a metamorphosis at the moment . . . it is going through a midlife crisis actually [laughter] . . . It was mainly information based or we were dealing with the objective of finding speakers, finding resources for issues surrounding menopause. Now a lot of it was in a medical context. We were looking at

osteoporosis. We were looking at diet. We were looking at incontinence issues. We were looking at hysterectomies, HRT . . . After we had done the gamut of all those topics I was very keen to do some skill development with these women.

The skills to be developed were firmly defined for the women. Alternative skills were promoted in the context of an assumption that medical advice was irrelevant:

> We were looking at workshops and we did workshops on massage, t'ai chi, personal development stuff like, self-esteem, confidence and that sort of thing . . . Women are saying . . . 'Look we are sick and tired of having hormones shoved in our faces. We are sick and tired of being told to go on a holiday when we can't afford to buy a pair of shoes.' That is not the answer. I think women have always been made to have a sort of like . . . 'You solve the problem!' . . . We wanted to then provide them with some skills to practise and to take away with them.

The women still had to solve their own problems. The results were mixed:

> It is sort of like a ripple effect that has happened at the health centre. For instance the t'ai chi stuff. We did a two-hour workshop and we ended up having to do a pilot program here with fifteen women. The evaluation of that was quite interesting in that these were women who had never ever challenged their beliefs or values or whatever . . . We have done four programs this year and we have even got bookings for next year . . .

But one t'ai chi session was enough for most of the women; they told Rose they 'weren't practising it because they forgot or the usual things'. A room was found where they could practise on their own and together as a group, but she is unsure if they do. Meanwhile, a residual group from several other initiatives meets at the centre. Rose reflects on what has been created, proud of it but not sure that it addresses the original goals:

> There are people that sort of stayed on from a gentle exercise program and it is all just like knitting into this huge yarn if you know what I mean. It is like a quilting effect what is happening . . . It is very complex now and that is why I think we are at a midlife crisis because we are not clear about the objectives of the group anymore . . . We

have gone from all that very clear information base to an — I mean in some ways it is probably meant to go that way.

She sees the groups as making sense in terms of a 'broader community-health philosophy' offering choice to the women who did stay:

> They are looking beyond what is currently available in terms of their doctors and the information around and now there is just so much. As I say, it is just like forming this huge blanket of stuff all intertwining with one another . . . if people have more options and choices then they seem to have . . . a lot more skills to be able to call on when they are feeling that perhaps they need some support.

Conclusion

Like the data from doctors, these accounts from community level providers fit oddly with the stereotypes of professional perspectives on women's health and menopause. The two bodies of data both confirmed the influence of that stereotype (it appeared in the accounts from professionals and those they talked to), and indicated the importance of questioning it. From this very complex data, a few conclusions are justified.

The ideal role presented in the literature for community health providers is adopted by very few. Some, but only some, advisers at the grass-roots level are giving a different sort of advice from that given by some (but not all) doctors. The contrast is no clearer than that.

However some themes occur *only* in the accounts at the community level, although never in a majority of those accounts. Only there did we hear the discourse of wellness and the emphasis on the naturalness of transition and ageing, and acceptance of 'natural' treatments (and sometimes pushing of them). Only at that level did advisers stress relationships with the 'whole woman'. Only there was there emphasis on taking time and listening, on ethnic and cultural diversity, and group interaction. Their approach to knowledge was different, only there did we meet the urgency (and sometimes uncritical urging) of information provision, and uncritical acceptance of anecdotal or personal experience as data. And only at the community level did we hear the message that you are 'responsible for your health' with the adviser as partner in this process. No doctor's account fitted the model presented at the start of this chapter, but it did fit the practice of a few community level advisers.

Overall, the data offer no support for assertions that there is a clear dichotomy between the biomedical and grass-roots, community level or nursing perspective. Clearly some community level advisers work with this dichotomy, but most work collaboratively in some way with medical advisers.

While for many women understanding of their midlife health depends on the 'private' relationship with their doctors, information provision at the community level is active and increasing. For some women it provides a source of wanted, informed decision-making. For more it usually offers a once-off chance to gather answers, fairly anonymously (no community interaction involved), to questions they find difficult to ask.

A number of factors strongly influence the availability of information and advice at the community level. These include demographic features of the local area: age distribution, women's workforce participation, ethnic diversity and resources. Our data suggest the importance of individual agents, energetic nurses and enthusiastic converts to community level nursing, some of whom promoted a series of events and processes affecting very many midlife women. The contributing factors in their role may be items of personal history or professional orientation. This is one of many reasons why the process of social construction of menopause is, for at least some women, startlingly local. Nothing in the literature, or the early group interviews, warned us of this possible factor. Middle-class and educated women we interviewed had usually only sought advice from the local general pratitioner. Community level advice was offered in very localised events.

Neither model of health practice offers a good account of what actually happened to most, let alone all, women. In particular, issues of power in both models deserve far greater attention. Many doctors appeared oblivious to the ways they wielded authority and assumed it would be obeyed. Equally, many advisers at the grassroots level simply assumed that information provision is empowering and ignored their own exercise of power in selecting what was provided. Advisers from both levels often treated information as a commodity, paying little attention to their own exercise of power in providing or withholding it, or to processes by which women acquire and use information.

Where doctors were least helpful, it was because they assumed they could offer just the information needed, and their authority was enough to reassure women that they need not know more. Grass-roots advisers made the opposite assumption, that women should be presented with information about everything that could come upon them in midlife, and every (ideologically acceptable) option, and then be left to figure out for themselves what was relevant and what they should do about it. Given this choice between authoritatively selected information and mass informing, many women reasonably opted to have decisions made for them, accompanied by only the information supporting that decision. In doing so, they of course reaffirmed the authority of the doctor.

Perhaps the most important message from this data is that both the health professionals and the women they advise are active participants in constructing advisers' roles, and thereby the knowledge women have access to, what they do with it and the processes by which they construct understandings of their lives.

POSTSCRIPT

This book is the result of a collaborative project, and working on it has been a rich and rewarding experience. When we started the project we had no idea where it would take us. We went into it with different versions of taken-for-granted assumptions about midlife and menopause. Almost all of these were challenged. We learned a lot from the women who shared their stories with us and made this book. We learned that menopause and midlife can be appalling experiences for a few, barely noticed by others, and between these two extremes the experiences were so varied that no stereotypes fitted them all. We learned that for most women, menopause and midlife offered an interval in the ongoing drama of their lives and that they were active agents in shaping that drama.

To uncover the variety of experiences and to throw the stereotypes in doubt is both confusing and enlightening. Menopause pictured, on the one hand, as an irrevocable Change of Life, attended by unattractive and unhappy images, was to be dreaded and survived. Menopause pictured, on the other hand, as liberating and the beginning of a stage of wisdom and peace was equally implausible. Not one woman we talked to fitted these extremes.

Women navigated midlife and menopause in individual ways, challenging the stereotypes and making sense of conflicting advice. For a significant majority menopause heralded a period of reassessment. The metaphor of intermission helped us make sense of the variety of ways women reported their responses to midlife and menopause. For some women this intermission was marked by a period of confusion, for others it was used as a period of 'time out' to reassess their goals and clear up unfinished business. Unfinished business included relationships with husbands, with parents, particularly mothers, and with children.

This book is not the definitive text and will not tell you all you need to know about midlife and menopause. However, we doubt that any one book can meet everyone's needs. What this book does represent is the experiences of a wide cross-section of Australian women. We recognise that they do not represent all women. Our sample was self-selected, and it does not represent many groups, for instance non-English speaking and lesbian women, the very poor and the very powerful. But those who chose to talk with us spoke openly and in detail of their midlives. We hope that hearing about others' experiences can help you make sense of your own, and that finding patterns across a variety of experiences can help predict and explain what is happening to you. It did for us.

If this is a stage of life you are curious about and you would like more information, the list of information and support services on page 229 provides details of an agency in each state that can offer help and advice.

INFORMATION AND SUPPORT SERVICES

For further information please contact:

Canberra
Women's Centre for Health Matters
Building 1, Pearce Centre
Collett Place
Pearce 2607
Information line (02) 6286 2043

New South Wales
Department for Women
Women's Information and Referral Service
Level 11, 100 Williams Street
Woolloomooloo 2011
(02) 9334 1160
Toll free 1800 817 227;
TTY 1800 673 304

Northern Territory
Community Health Centre
Territory Health Services
Flynn Drive, Gillen Area
(08) 8951 6711

Queensland
Women's Health Centre Inc. Brisbane
165 Gregory Terrace
Spring Hill 4004
(07) 3839 9988
Information line 1800 017 676
TTY (07) 3831 5508

South Australia
Women's Health Statewide
64 Pennington Terrace
North Adelaide 5006
(08) 8267 5366
Women's Health Line 1800 182 098

Tasmania
Hobart's Women's Health Centre
326 Elizabeth Street
North Hobart 7000
(03) 6231 3212

Victoria
Women's Health Victoria (formerly known as Healthsharing Women's Health Resource Service)
Queen Victoria Women's Centre
210 Lonsdale Street
Melbourne 3000
Women's Health Line 1800 133 321

Western Australia
Health Information Resource Service
King Edward Memorial Hospital
374 Bagot Road
Subiaco 6008
(08) 9340 1100
Toll free 1800 651 100

Please note that these telephone numbers incorporate all AUSTEL's planned changes to Australian telephone numbers up until August 1997.

NOTES

1 Introduction
1. The original project was funded for three years by the National Health and Medical Research Foundation and Victorian Health Promotions Foundation. La Trobe University provided smaller-scale funding during the project. The Risk Perception Project was funded by the Australian Research Council.

2 Women's images of menopause
1. All comparisons with Australian figures are based on 1992 Australian Bureau of Statistics figures as these correspond to the period in which the survey was conducted.

3 Mirrors of menopause: The popular literature
1. With regard to menopause as a hidden experience rather than a taboo subject, Sophy Laws (1990) refers to the notion of etiquette in relation to menstruation — which may well hold true for menopause.
2. The *Australian Women's Weekly* published articles or medical columns with menopause as the focus in June 1986, December 1986, May 1989 and November 1990; *Family Circle* in April 1988, January 1989, May 1989, 1990 and November 1991; *Ita* in April 1989, May 1989, January 1990, August 1990, September 1990, December 1990, July 1991, October 1991 and October 1992; *Woman's Day* in March 1992; and *New Woman* in April 1992.
3. References included *The Change* by Germaine Greer, Llewellyn-Jones and Abraham's *Everywoman's Middle Years*, *Ourselves Growing Older* produced by The Boston Women's Collective, *Older Women Ready or Not* by Louise Anike and Lynette Arial, *Overcoming the Menopause Naturally* by Caroline Shreeve,

Menopause without Medicine by Linda Ojeda, and *Menopause: You Can Give It a Miss!* by Sandra Cabot.
4   Research is being done at Melbourne University by S. Skelly into the efficacy of Chinese herbs for relief of menopausal symptoms. Reported in *Hospital Quarterly*, Nov/Dec 1995, pp. 73–9.
5   There is some evidence to suggest that the protective effect of oestrogen on the cardiovascular system may be negated by the use of progesterone (progestogens) aimed at preventing cancer of the uterus (Goldman & Tosteson 1991).

Studies showing a link between breast cancer and HRT, most particularly oestrogen alone, started to appear in the mid-1980s. A meta-analysis by Sillero-Arenas, Delgado-Rodriguez, Rodigues-Canteras, Bueno-Cavanillas and Galve Vargas (1992) of 37 original studies of breast cancer risk revealed a small but statistically significant relative risk of 1.06. Women who experienced natural menopause seemed to have a slightly higher (1.13) risk. A nonsignificant increasing trend was found between duration of hormone therapy and breast cancer risk.

While evidence associating HRT with an increased risk of breast cancer is growing, more studies need to be done showing a clear link between the use of combined oestrogen and progesterone, the length of therapy and cancer of the breast. The first study to demonstrate a link between combined oestrogen and progesterone (progestin) therapy and breast cancer was reported by Bergkvist et al. (1989). Women using preparations combining both oestrogen and progestin for more than 6 years had a higher rate of breast cancer (4 times higher than non-users) than women using oestrogen alone (two times higher than non-users).

4   The body in midlife
1   Discourse is defined as both an act of communication through language and as statements governed by rules and having social and political power, for example, medical discourse.

5   Making the change
1   In a conversation with Anselm Strauss I queried the absence of agency in the writing on status passage. He observed that this might be because the concept had been born in a study of dying, a study that focused on the people around the patient. Elsewhere he had written more about ways people maintain a sense of continuity through changes, how they put their lives together linguistically, practically, even when lives may be 'split' — as with migrants. 'Did menopause SPLIT women's lives?' he asked. I pointed out that women called it the Change, but from that conversation I was alerted to the difference between changed lives and split lives.

7   Private parts in public places
1   Women aged 40–55 comprised 65% of the female workforce

compared with 37% in 1966 (Australian Bureau of Statistics 1993).

9   **What *did* the doctor say?**
1   Many methodological issues are involved here. Observation of consultations is clearly problematic in areas where only a very few clinicians will grant permission. The data from such observations have to be interpreted as records of performances in which the lead actor, the physician, is highly aware of the audience and possible interpretations in research reports. Hence observation studies restricted to once-off attendance at clinical encounters will be highly unlikely to be either useful or ethical, given the intimate nature of the issues for a woman, and the ideological and political debates surrounding HRT. On the other hand, interpretations of past encounters, by the woman or the clinician, necessarily present only one of several possible interpretations and partial recall.

REFERENCES

Anike, L. & Ariel, L. (1987). *Older Women Ready or Not.* L. Anike & L. Ariel, Sydney.
Anon (1988). Skin care feature (citing role models). *Australian Women's Weekly*, March.
Armstrong, Diane (1990). 'Midlife crisis the getting of wisdom'. *Ita*, May.
Ashcroft, M. D. & O'Brien, D. (1992). 'Broadmeadows Community Health Services Menopause Clinic'. *Healthsharing Women's Research Issues Forum 11: Hormone Replacement Therapy*, April.
Australian Bureau of Statistics (1993). Catalogue no. 411300. *Women in Australia*. Canberra.
Ballinger, S. & Walker, W. (1987). *Not the Change of Life: Breaking the Menopause Taboo*. Penguin, Melbourne.
Barker, Vic (1990). 'Osteoporosis the unnecessary disease'. *Ita*, January.
Bart, P. B. & Grossman, M. (1978). 'Menopause'. In *Sexual and Reproductive Aspects of Women's Health Care*, eds M. T. Notman & C. Nadelson. Plenum, New York.
Baum, F., Fry, D. & Lennie, I. (1992). *Community Health, Policy and Practice in Australia*. Pluto Press, Sydney.
Beard, M. & Curtis, L. (1988). *Menopause and the Years Ahead*. Fisher Books, Tuscon, Arizona.
Beasley, Margo (1989). 'Menopause. Women's health in the 90s'. *Australian Women's Weekly*, May.
Beaumont, Janise (1990). 'A tale of two face lifts'. *Ita*, May.
Bell, S. E. (1986). 'A new model of medical technological development: A case study of DES'. *Research in the Sociology of Health Care*, vol. 4, pp. 1–32.
Bell, S. E. (1987). 'Changing ideas: The medicalisation of menopause'. *Social Science and Medicine*, vol. 24, pp. 535–42.

Bennett, D. & Degeling, D. (1988). *Midlife—it's OK*. Bay Books, Sydney.
Bergkvist, L., Adami, H-O., Persson, I., Hoover, R. & Schairer, C. (1989). 'The risk of breast cancer after estrogens and estrogen/progestin replacement'. *New England Journal of Medicine*, vol. 321, pp. 293–7.
Beyenne, Y. (1986). 'Cultural significance and physiological manifestations of menopause: A biocultural analysis'. *Culture, Medicine and Psychiatry*, vol. 10, pp. 47–71.
Bordieu, P. (1992). *The Logic of Practice*. Polity Press, Cambridge.
Bordo, S. (1992). 'Anorexia nervosa: psychopathology as crystallization of culture'. In *Knowing Women: Feminism and Knowledge*, eds H. Crowley & S. Himmelweit. Polity Press, Cambridge.
Brinton, L. A. & Fraumeni, J. F. (1986). 'Epidemiology of uterine cervical cancer'. *Journal of Chronic Diseases*, vol. 39, p. 1051.
Bromwich, P. (1989). *Menopause: Treating the Symptoms*. British Medical Association, Wellingborough.
Broom, D. (1991). *Damned If We Do: Contradictions in Women's Health*. Allen & Unwin, Sydney.
Cabot, S. (1989). 'Osteoporosis the silent epidemic'. *Ita*, April.
Cabot, S. (1991). *Menopause: You Can Give It a Miss!* Women's Health Advisory Service, Melbourne.
Cabot, Sandra, Wilson, Mary Joe & Garratt, Elizabeth (1989). 'The menopause and how it will affect you'. *Ita*, May.
Cohen, Sherry (1991). 'Sex gets better as you get older'. *New Woman*, October.
Coney, S. (1993). *The Menopause Industry: A Guide to Medicine's Discovery of the Mid-life Woman*. Spinifex, Melbourne.
Cooke, D. J. & Greene, J. G. (1981). 'Types of life events in relation to symptoms at the climacterium'. *Journal of Psychosomatic Research*, vol. 25, pp. 5–11.
Coope, J. & Marsh, J. (1992). 'Can we improve compliance with long-term HRT?' *Maturitas*, vol. 15, pp. 151–8.
Coward, R. (1983). *Patriarchal Precedents: Sexuality and Social Relations*. Routledge & Kegan Paul, London.
Coward, S. (1984). *Female Desire*. Paladin, London.
Daly, J., Miller, R. & Richards, L. (1992). Social construction of menopause, a qualitative approach. Australian Menopause Conference, Melbourne.
Datan, N. (1986). 'Corpses, lepers and menstruating women: Tradition, transition and the sociology of knowledge'. *Sex Roles*, vol. 14, no. 12.
Davis, D. L. (1986). 'The meaning of menopause in a Newfoundland fishing village'. *Culture, Medicine and Psychiatry*, vol. 10, pp. 23–46.
Dee, Ho (1994). 'The no drug menopause'. *Australian Women's Weekly*, September.
Dennerstein, L., Smith, A., Morse, C., Burger, H., Greem, A., Hopper, J. & Ryan, M. (1993). 'Menopausal symptoms in Australian women'. *Medical Journal of Australia*, vol. 159, pp. 232–6.
Dervin, B. & Nilan, M. (1986). 'Information needs and uses'. In *Annual*

Review of Information Science and Technology, vol. 21, ed. M. E. Williams. Knowledge Industry Publications for the American Society for Information Science, Medford, NJ.

Dickson, A. & Henriques, N. (1988). *Women on Menopause: A Practical Guide to a Positive Transition.* Healing Arts Press, Rochester.

Dickson, G. L. (1990). 'A feminist poststructuralist analysis of the knowledge of menopause'. *Advances in Nursing Science*, vol.12, no. 3, pp. 15–31.

do Rozario, L. (1994). 'Wellness perspectives in community work: Towards an ecological and transformational model of practice'. In *Primary Health Care, the Way to the Future*, ed. C. Cooney. Prentice Hall, Sydney.

Donovan, J. C. (1951). 'The menopausal syndrome: A study of case histories'. *American Journal of Obstetrics and Gynaecology*, vol. 62, pp. 1281–91.

Doress, P. D. & Siegal, D. L. (1987). *Ourselves growing older.* Simon & Schuster, New York.

Downing, C. (1991). *Journey through Menopause: A Personal Rite of Passage.* Crossroads, New York.

Edison, Joan (1988). 'Challenging the myths of menopause'. *Family Circle*, 17 April.

Ettinger, B., Genant, H. & Cann, C. (1985). 'Long-term estrogen replacement therapy prevents bone loss and fractures'. *Annals of Internal Medicine*, vol. 102, pp. 319–24.

Ewertz, M. (1988). 'Influence of non-contraceptive exogenous and endogenous sex hormones on breast cancer risk in Denmark'. *International Journal of Cancer*, vol. 42, pp. 832–8.

Firestone, S. (1970). *The Dialectic of Sex: The Case for Feminist Revolution.* William Morrow, New York. (Paladin, London, 1972.)

Foucault, M. (1980). 'Power/knowledge, selected interviews and other writings'. Pantheon Books, New York.

Foucault, M. (1981). *The History of Sexuality Volume 1: An Introduction.* Pelican, Harmondsworth.

Gambrell, R. D. (1986). 'Prevention of endometrial cancer with progestogen'. *Maturitas*, vol. 8, pp. 159–68.

Gannon, L. R. (1985). *Menstrual Disorders and Menopause: Biological, Psychological and Cultural Research.* Praegar, New York.

Giddens, A. (1991). *Modernity and Self-Identity: Self and Society in the Late Modern Age.* Polity Press, Cambridge.

Goffman, E. (1971). *Relations in Public.* Allen Lane, London.

Goldman, L. & Tosteson, A. N. A. (1991). 'Uncertainty about post menopausal estrogen: Time for action not debate'. *New England Journal of Medicine*, vol. 315, no. 11, pp. 800–20.

Greenwood, S. (1989). *Menopause Naturally: Preparing for the Second Half of Life.* Volcano Press, San Francisco.

Greer, G. (1970). *The Female Eunuch.* Paladin, London.

Greer, G. (1991). *The Change: Women, Ageing and the Menopause.* Hamish Hamilton, London.

Gross, Amy (1991). 'You are only as old as you feel'. *New Woman*, April.
Guillemin, M. (1994). Whose menopause? Women's experiences and technologies in the menopause clinic. Paper to The Australian Sociological Association (TASA) Conference, Deakin University, December.
Hailes, J. (1986). *The Middle Years*. Pitman, Melbourne.
Harper, Helen (1991). 'All in the family'. *Ita*, November.
Harper, J. & Richards, L. (1986). *Mothers and Working Mothers*. Rev. edn. Penguin, Melbourne.
Hershon, Oelanie (1991). 'Boning up on osteoporosis'. *Ita*, July.
Hollway, W. (1984). 'Gender differences and the production of subjectivity'. In *Changing the Subject: Psychology, Social Regulation and Subjectivity*, eds J. Henriques et al. Methuen, London.
Hunt, L. (1991). The women's health movement: A study of a solution. Paper presented to The Australian Sociological Association (TASA) Conference, Perth, December.
Hunter, M. (1990). *Your Menopause: Prepare Now for a Positive Future*. Pandora, London.
Kaufert, P. (1982). 'Myth and the Menopause'. *Sociology of Health and Illness*, vol. 4, pp. 141–66.
Kaufert, P.A. (1986). 'Menstruation and menstrual change: Women in midlife'. *Health Care for Women International*, vol. 7, pp. 1–2, 63–76.
Kaufert, P.A. & Gilbert, P. (1986). 'Women, menopause, and medicalization'. *Culture, Medicine and Psychiatry*, vol. 10, March, pp. 7–21.
Kearsley, E. (1989). 'Menopause — your questions answered'. *Family Circle*, 28 May.
Kearsley, E. (1990). *Female Menopause: A Personal Experience*. E. Kearsley, Hobart.
Kennedy, Heather (1990). 'Eat well to be well'. *Family Circle*, October.
Kerr, Susan (1990). 'Facing menopause with confidence', *Family Circle*, 17 June.
Laws, S. (1990). *Issues of Blood*. Macmillan, London.
Lewis, Cathy (1996). Location, women and menopause. A report submitted to the authors' Menopause Project, October.
Llewellyn-Jones, D. (1989). *Everywoman: A Gynaecological Guide to Life*. Faber, London.
Llewellyn-Jones, D. & Abraham, S. (1988). *Menopause*. Penguin, Melbourne.
Llewellyn-Jones, D. & Abraham, S. (1992). *Everywoman's Middle Years*. Ashwood House Medical, Melbourne.
Lock, M. (1982). 'Models and practice in medicine: Menopause as syndrome or life transition?' *Culture, Medicine and Psychiatry*, vol. 6, no. 3, pp. 261–80.
Lock, M. (1985). 'Models and practice in medicine: Menopause as syndrome or life transition?' In *Physicians of Western Medicine:*

Anthropological Approaches to Theory and Practice, eds R. S. Hahn & A.D. Gaines. Reidel, Boston.
Logothetis, M. L. (1991). 'Our legacy: Medical views of the menopausal woman.' In *Women of the 14th Moon: Writings on Menopause*, eds D. Taylor & A. Coverdale Sumrall. The Crossing Press, Freedom.
Lord, Vicki (1989). 'Confident looks at any age'. *Ita*, April.
Magazines 2000 (1996). Magazines: You can't put them down. An information sheet produced as part of a Magazines 2000 Initiative. Mag1314\A.
Mankovitz, A. (1984). *Change of Life: A Psychological Study of Dreams and the Menopause*. Inner City Books, Toronto.
Martin, E. (1987). *The Woman in the Body: A Cultural Analysis of Reproduction*. Beacon Press, Boston.
Maseide, P. (1991). 'Possibly abusive, often benign and always necessary: On power and domination in medical practice'. *Sociology of Health and Illness*, vol. 13, no. 4, pp. 545–61.
May, C. (1992). 'Individual care? Power and Subjectivity in therapeutic relationships'. *Sociology*, vol. 26, no. 4, pp. 589–602.
McCrea, F. (1983). 'The politics of menopause: The discovery of a deficiency disease'. *Social Problems*, vol. 31, no. 1, pp. 111–23.
McDarra, Fiona (1989). 'Update on osteoporosis'. *Family Circle*, 1 January.
McKenzie, Frances (1986). 'Boning up on osteoporosis'. *Australian Women's Weekly*, December.
McKenzie, Frances (1990). 'Healthwise: Good health during and after menopause'. *Australian Women's Weekly*, November.
McPherson, K.I. (1981). 'Menopause as disease: The social construction of a metaphor'. *Advances in Nursing Science*, vol. 3, no. 2, pp. 95–113.
McPherson, K.I. (1992). 'Cardiovascular disease in women and non contraceptive use of hormones: A feminist analysis'. *Advances in Nursing Science*, vol. 14, no. 4, pp. 34–9.
McPherson, K.I. (1985). 'Osteoporosis and menopause: A feminist analysis of the social construction of a syndrome'. *Advances in Nursing Science*, vol. 7, no. 4, pp. 11–22.
Moore, H. (1994). *A Passion for Difference*. Polity Press, Cambridge.
Morse, Carol (1990). 'Bone update'. *Ita*, December.
Murphy, S. M. (1983). *The Midlife Wanderer: The Woman Religious in Midlife Transition*. Mercantile Printing, Massachusetts.
O'Toole, R. & O'Toole, A.W. 'Menopause: Analysis of a status passage'. *Free Inquiry in Creative Sociology*, vol. 16, no. 1, pp. 85–91.
Oaks, Wendy (1991). 'HRT: Latest thoughts on beating the change of life'. *Ita*, April.
Oakley, A. (1980). *Woman Confined: Towards a Sociology of Child Birth*. Martin Robertson, Oxford.
Ojeda, L. (1989). *Menopause without Medicine*. Hunter House, Claremont.
Parsons, C. D. F. & Buckenham, J. (1991). 'Let's be reasonable: Health promotion and health screening'. *Shaping Nursing Theory and*

Practice Conference Proceedings, La Trobe University, Melbourne, October.
Parsons, C. D. F. & Wakely, P. (1991). 'Idioms of distress: Somatic responses to distress in everyday life'. *Culture, Medicine and Psychiatry*, vol. 15, pp. 111–32.
Phillips, A. & Raskussen, J. (1985). *The New Our Bodies Ourselves: A Health Book for and by Women*. Penguin, Harmondsworth.
Pogrebin, Letty Cottin (1989). 'Turning 50 and panicking'. *New Woman*, November.
Polit, D. & LaRocco, S. A. (1980). 'Social and psychological correlates of menopausal symptoms'. *Psychosomatic Medicine*, vol. 42, no. 3, pp. 335–45.
Posner, J. (1979). 'It's all in your head: Feminist and medical models of menopause (strange bedfellows)'. *Sex Roles*, vol. 5, no. 2, pp. 179–90.
Post Registration (Nursing) Education Advisory Committee (1991). *Great Expectations of the Community Health Nurse: Community Health Nurses Study*, June.
Powell, Robin (1991). 'A change for the better'. *Family Circle*, November.
Reitz, R. (1987). *Menopause a Positive Approach*. Unwin, London.
Rich, A. (1977). *Of Women Born*. Virago, London.
Richards, L. (1995). 'Transition work! Reflections on a three year NUD•IST project'. In *Computing and Qualitative Research Studies in Qualitative Methodology*, vol. 5, ed. R. G. Burgess. JAI Press, London.
Richards, L. & Richards, T. J. (1991a). 'Computing in qualitative analysis: A healthy development?' *Qualitative Health Research*, vol. 1, pp. 234–62.
Richards, L. & Richards, T. J. (1991b). 'The transformation of qualitative method: Computational paradigms and research processes'. In *Using Computers in Qualitative Research*, eds N. G. Fielding & R. M. Lee. Sage Publications, Newbury Park, CA.
Richards, L. & Richards, T. J. (1995). 'From filing cabinet to computer'. In *Analysing Qualitative Data*, eds R.W. Burgess & A. Bryman. Routledge, London.
Richards, T. J. & Richards, L. (1994). 'Using computers in qualitative analysis'. In *Handbook of Qualitative Research*, eds N. K. Denzin & Yvonna S. Lincoln. Sage Publications, Newbury Park, CA.
Riggs, L. B. & Melton, L. J. (1986). 'Involutional osteoporosis'. *New England Journal of Medicine*, vol. 314, no. 36, pp. 1676–86.
Rorden, J. W. & McLennan, J. (1992). *Community Health Nursing, Theory and Practice*. Harcourt Brace Jovanovich, Sydney.
Ross, R. K., Paganini-Hill, A., Mack, T. M. & Henderson, B. E. (1987). 'Estrogen use and cardiovascular disease'. In *Menopause, Physiology and Pharmacology*, ed. D. R. Mishell Jr. Yearbook, Chicago, pp. 209–24.
Ruben, L. B. (1979). *Women of a Certain Age: The Midlife Search for Self*. Harper & Row, New York.

Saltman, D. (1994). *In Transition: A Guide to Menopause.* Choice Books, Sydney.
Segal, L. (1992). 'Sensual uncertainty, or why the clitoris is not enough'. In *Knowing Women: Feminism and Knowledge,* eds H. Crowley & S. Himmelweit. Polity Press, Cambridge.
Seibold, C., Richards, L. & Simon, D. (1994). 'Feminist method and qualitative research about midlife'. *Journal of Advanced Nursing,* vol. 19, pp. 394–402.
Sheehy, G. (1993). *The Silent Passage: Menopause.* Fontana, London.
Shreeve, C. M. (1986). *Overcoming the Menopause Naturally.* Arrow, London.
Sillero-Arenas, M., Delgado-Rodriguez, M., Rodigues-Canteras, R., Bueno-Cavanillas, A. & Galve Vargas, R. (1992). 'Menopausal hormone replacement therapy and breast cancer: A meta-analysis'. *Obstetrics and Gynecology,* vol. 79, pp. 286–94.
Simon, D. (1994). The doctor's dilemma: An inquiry into the relationship between general practitioners and their patients. Honours thesis, La Trobe University.
Singh, S. (1993). Marriage, money and information: Australian consumers' use of banks. PhD thesis, La Trobe University.
Smith, D. C., Prentice, R., Thompson, J. & Herrman W. L. (1975). 'Association of exogenous estrogen and endometrial cancer'. *New England Journal of Medicine,* vol. 293, pp. 1164–7.
Strauss, A.L. (1987). *Qualitative Analysis for Social Scientists.* Cambridge University Press, Cambridge, MA.
Strauss, A.L. & Corbin, J. (1990). *Basics of Qualitative Research, Grounded Theory Procedures and Techniques.* Sage Publications, London.
Taylor, D. & Coverdale Sumrall, A. (1991). *Women of the 14th Moon: Writings on Menopause.* The Crossing Press, Freedom.
Turner, B. (1987). *Medical Power and Social Knowledge.* Sage Publications, London.
Turner, Bunty (1990). 'The good news about osteoporosis: It can be prevented'. *Ita,* August.
Wangman, Suzanne (1988). 'Glamour for a busy grandmother'. *Australian Women's Weekly,* July.
Weisser, Hilary (1991). 'Hormone replacement: The questions you want to ask and the answers'. *Ita,* October.
Wilson, R.A. (1966). *Feminine Forever.* W. H. Allen, London.
Zeil, H. & Finkle, W. (1975). 'Increased risk of endometrial cancer among users of conjugated estrogens'. *New England Journal of Medicine,* vol. 293, pp. 1167–70.

INDEX

abortion 54, 55, 65, 97
aching and creaking joints 106, 108, 209
advice
   from community level health-care advisers 199–225
   from medical carers 171–98
   from mothers 83–85
   from other women 38
age
   and anxiety 136
   and images of menopause 25–7
age distribution, of respondents 16
ageing 123, 125
   acceptance of 72, 73, 210
   and the body 69–70, 72–3, 109
   fear of 89
   HRT to prevent premature 182
   negative images of 45, 131
   positive images of 120
agency 94, 95, 98
alternative healers, trust in 169
alternative health model 42–3, 44–6
alternative therapies 36, 40–1, 47, 63, 98

tolerance by community carers of 210–11
see also herbal remedies; naturopathy
anonymity of surveyed population 6, 14–15
athletic body 70
attractiveness
   and age 68–9, 75
   importance of 67
awareness of the body 51–2
avoiding change 93–4

back problems 133
beauty myth 37, 72, 210
becoming old *see* ageing
'been through' menopause 86
biological destiny 123–4
biological determinism 66–7, 74
biomedical model
   as backdrop only 195
   critical stereotype 175–89
   in the literature 35, 42, 43
   inadequacy of evidence for 172–4
   interpretation 195–8

INDEX

poor fit with data 36, 178–89
blood tests 58
body
  and ageing 69–70, 72–3
  anthropological view 70–1
  as problematic 49–50
  awareness of the 51
  controlling the 54–62, 96, 99
  listening to the 62–4
  out of control 51–2, 90–1
  physical attractiveness of the 67, 68–9, 75
  pre-menopausal 49–51, 54–7, 65–6
  understanding in a sexual way 67–8
  viewing the 64–73
  working the 50–4
  see also mind–body divide
books
  as source of information and reassurance 38–9
  on menopause 37–8
breast cancer 37, 60, 119, 159, 166
  and long-term HRT use 59–60
  and trust in healer's advice 168
  inherited 157–8
  see also mammogram
burn-out 51, 114

Cabot, Sandra 37, 38
  emphasis on HRT 40
calcium in menopause treatment 34, 36, 180, 181, 216
cancer
  threats of 166, 168
  see also specific cancers, e.g. breast cancer
cardiovascular disease, prevention through HRT 20, 35, 44
care
  community health carers' attitudes to 205–11
  doctors' attitudes to 176–7, 179–83
career, in midlife 135–6
caring role of women
  for children 98, 135, 142, 146
  for elderly parents 92, 110, 143–4

pre-midlife 120
cervical cancer 149, 158, 159
  prevention through Pap smear 163
cessation of menses *see* menstruation
'Change, the' 77, 84, 88, 104
changing attitudes
  to menopause 28–31, 128–9
  to women 66, 103
childhood memories 107, 108, 109, 115, 120
childlessness, regrets at midlife of 123–4
children 16, 98, 123–4, 135, 142, 146
colon cancer 166
community education campaigns 100, 101, 102
community health nurses
  approach to discussing menopause with women 216–17
  as watchdogs in monitoring medical advice 207, 208
  attitude to hormone treatment 208–9
  establishment of women's groups on menopause 205, 212
  information sessions on menopause 205, 214, 215
  menopause seen in 'total context' 212
  role 200–1, 223
  untapped as resource by respondents 203
community-level health care
  and power 218, 220
  and wellness 209–10
  attitudes to alternative care 210–11
  attitudes to medical care 205, 206–7
  caring function 205–9
  claims for 200–2
  factors influencing availability of information 224
  holistic approach to menopause services 201
  HRT as contentious issue 207–9
  information and empowerment 217–20, 225

irrelevance to respondents 203–5
knowledge transfer on menopause-
    related issues 215–18
listening and spending time with
    women 213–14, 223
menopause clinics 205–6
model 201–2
recommends women make their
    own choice over HRT 208
referrals to general practitioners
    205, 207
relationship with the 'whole
    person' 211–13, 223
relationships with women
    211–15
settings for information sessions
    214–15
talks on menopause 212
telephone interviews with carers
    3, 203–4
variation in menopausal
    information available 204–5
see also rural community health
    care
companionship at work 130, 140
Coney, S. 43
confidence in self 52, 130, 145,
    153
contraceptive pill 21, 54–5, 56, 57,
    180–1
controlling the body 54–62, 96,
    107
    following hysterectomy 99
    in midlife 57–62, 138

data handling 7–8
depression
    during menopause 42, 62, 123
    while on progesterone 64
diary keeping 49
diet 34, 36, 71, 216
disease prevention, and screening
    162–4
disease threat, as motivation for
    screening 166–7
distress 52, 62
divorced women in midlife 48–9,
    67
doctors see medical carers
drug companies 44, 182, 193

dry skin 102, 107

embarrassment
    from forgetfulness 53–4
    from hot flushes 56
    over flooding 56, 138
    over screening 164
emotional lability 53, 97, 135
employment opportunities, and
    ageing 136
employment status, of respondents
    16
empowerment 101–3, 213, 215,
    217–18, 220
    see also taking charge; time out;
        women
empty nest 91–3, 153
endometrial cancer 44
endometriosis 72
energy
    demands on 131, 136
    lack of 105, 135, 138
erratic behaviour 118–19, 120
ethics of group interviews 2
ethnicity of respondents 15–16
exercise 216
    and body image 69–70
    in menopause treatment 34, 36

face-to-face interviews 5
family
    and work 131, 134–5, 138,
        142–4, 146, 147
    as private sphere 129
    changing roles 129, 131, 142–4
    load for midlife women 43,
        142–4
family medical history, as natural
    risk 156–8, 169–70
fatalism 95
fecundity, loss of 57, 88
feminist writing
    on biological determinism 66–7,
        74
    on contraception 54–5
    on discourses of body 50
    on HRT 59–60
    on menopause 25, 28, 41, 44–5,
        56, 102
    on mind–body divide 73–6

on patriarchal family 75, 103
on sexuality 68
on treatment of menopause 34, 45–6, 62, 74, 104
fertility control 54–7
financial rewards of work 130–1
fitness
 and body image 69–70
 of respondents 17
flooding 56, 58, 138
forgetfulness 53–4, 102, 106, 118
Foucault, M. 57, 174–5
freedom
 associated with family stage 93
 associated with menopause 24–5
 following hysterectomy 96–7
friends, at work 139–42

general practitioners *see* medical carers
geographical distance, and network maintenance 140–1
'getting through' menopause 23, 83–7
'grass roots' health care *see* community-level health care
Greer, Germaine
 'crazy' image of menopausal women 41–2
 The Change 37–8, 39, 40–1, 43, 64, 107
group interviews 2–3, 4
gynaecological history of respondents 17
gynaecologists *see* medical carers

hair, changes 102
health education, community-based 213
health history, as reason for HRT 60
health prevention, through screening 17–18, 162–7
health professionals
 telephone interviews with 3, 203–4
 trust of 167–8
 used by respondents 18
 views on menopause treatments 35
 see also community-level health care

health promotion messages, misinterpretation of 163, 170
health risks
 and screening 162–4
 and self trust 167
 associated with midlife 156–62
 discourses 159–60
 from disease 166–7
 HRT for control 160–2
 natural 156–8
 statistical data 158–9, 167
 unnatural 158–60
health screening *see* screening
health status
 midlife women 19–21
 respondents 16–18
heart disease, threat of 166
herbal remedies 36, 63, 169
home, and paid work 127–8, 131
hormone replacement therapy *see* HRT
hormone therapy 20, 43, 138–9
hot flushes 51–2, 58, 91, 99, 100, 109, 114
 and embarrassment 56, 90
 as reason for taking HRT 61
 at work 126–7
 distress associated with 52, 98
HRT
 alternative health model in popular texts 42–3, 44–6
 and libido 61–2, 63–4, 181–2
 as a disease preventative 160–1, 170, 181–2
 as contentious issue in community health care 207–9
 as patient-specific 179, 183
 as treatment 160, 170
 biomedical model in popular texts 42, 43–4
 controversy over the medical evidence 186
 doctors' unwillingness to make decision 182, 185, 187
 doctors' views of safety 179–82
 doctors' views on taking 171, 179–80, 181–3
 dosage level difficulties 184–5
 for avoiding transition 93–4
 for cardiovascular disease

prevention   20, 35, 40, 44, 181
  for controlling the body   57,
    59–62, 75
  for osteoporosis prevention   20,
    34, 35, 40, 44, 61, 181, 188
  for premature ageing prevention
    182
  health risks with   34, 36, 59–60,
    101, 186
  physiological reaction to   193,
    194–5
  popular magazines support for
    34–6, 94, 192
  positive experiences with   64, 82
  reasons for cessation of   62–3, 98
  reasons for taking   59–60, 61,
    138–9
  resistance to   60–1, 94
  to control unnatural health risks
    160–2
  use by sample women   20, 59,
    160
  women's expected length of use
    20–1, 94
  women's right to choose   187–8,
    192–3
humiliation of a body out of control
  90
husband
  changing relationship   96, 100
  not often mentioned   84
  support from   91, 133, 142, 144
hysterectomy   17, 72, 88
  relief following   96, 97, 99

identity, concept of   124
illnesses and ailments   106, 113–14,
    115, 133
  see also specific conditions, e.g.
    osteoporosis
imagination   123
infertility, associated with
    menopause   23, 27
information about menopause
  access to information   32–3
  and empowerment   217–20
  see also support services
inherited health risks   156–8
intermission, menopause as   1, 9,
    77–104

interview methods   2–5, 48–9
intra-uterine contraceptive devices
    (IUDs)   54, 55
investment, notion of   75
irrational fears   114, 117–18, 122
irregular periods   58, 60, 112, 121

knowledge
  of medical carers   177, 185–6
  transfer through community health
    carers   215–18

large-scale survey   5–6, 13–31
libido see sexual desire
listening to the body   62–4
Llewellyn-Jones, Derek   38
  and Abraham, S., *Menopause* 39,
    40
  Everywoman   39
lung cancer   158

magazines   3, 33–7
  alternative therapies   36
  medical authorities' views in   35–6
  messages picked up from   33–4
  statistics on diseases and risks
    158–9, 167
  support for HRT   34–6, 94, 182
  women's use of information in
    46–7
mailed-out survey   5–6, 14
male-dominated medical profession
    172, 184, 186–7, 197
  resentment of   60, 74, 190–1
male-dominated world   108
mammogram   18, 37, 149, 165
marital status of respondents   16
marriage
  midlife changes   134
media health messages   169
medical advice
  women's attitude to   172,
    189–95
  women's resistance to over HRT
    60, 94, 98
medical carers
  advice from   171–98
  advice over HRT   171, 179–81
  advice to women about
    menopause, critics' view   175–6

advice to women about
  menopause, their view   178–89
and women's right to choose type
  of therapy 187–8
attitude to care   176–7, 179–83
community health attitude to
  205, 206–7
displeasure at outside sources of
  information   187, 198
disquiet at women's self-diagnosis
  187, 197
folk models   175
holistic view of patients   196
lack of respect towards patients
  60, 186
narrowly medical approach to
  treatment   179–80, 197
negative attitudes towards
  menopause   184
power and authority of   177,
  178, 187–9, 225
relationship to women patients
  177, 183–5, 187–9, 192–3, 198
scientific knowledge   177, 185–6
treatment orientation   181–2
trust of   167–8
uncertainty over HRT dosage
  levels and side-effects   184–5,
  198
views on menopause treatments
  35, 36–7
views on scientific evidence over
  HRT   186
see also biomedical model;
  community-level health care;
  health professionals
medical dominance   174–5
medical interaction, pragmatic model
  of (Maeside)   196, 197
medical texts
  coverage of menopause   174
memory   53–4
menopausal symptoms   19, 51–2,
  58, 90–1, 97–8, 100–3, 106,
  114, 209
  as unnatural health risk   161–2
  inappropriate treatment for   58–9
  management of at work 138–9
  see also specifics, e.g. hot flushes
menopausal treatments   20, 34–6,
  59–60, 72, 98–9
  see also specifics, e.g. HRT
menopause
  age and images of   25–7, 136
  and osteoporosis   34–5, 101
  and wellness   209–10
  and work   83, 98, 126, 132, 137
  anticipated physical and
    psychological changes 78–9,
    101, 152–3
  as a deficiency disease   34, 36,
    45, 176, 180–1
  as a medical issue   28, 39–40,
    176–7
  as a natural event   40
  as taboo subject   21, 25, 29, 31
  health advice   3
  images of 8, 21–8, 41, 86, 101,
    104, 152, 176–7, 226–7
  narrowly medical approach to care
    179–80
  one woman's diary   105–25
  words associated with   22–8
  see also specific topics
menstrual symptoms   50–1
menstruation
  as a status passage   88–9
  and control   74
  cessation of   19, 87–9
  irregularity of   60, 88, 112, 121
  positive aspects of   51, 96
  problems with   50–1, 64–5, 132
  secrecy about   50
mental decline   52–3, 123, 152–3,
  155, 209
midlife
  and personal health management
    153–4
  and women's health   149–70
  as life stage   91–3, 152
  as period of uncertainty 153–4
  in the 1990s   128–9
  'midlife crisis'   153
  sources of information about   33
  what does it mean?   154–6
  women's perceptions of   13,
    152–6
midlife health risks   155
  as natural and unnatural risks
    156–62

midlife risks   152–6
midlife women
 and health status   19–21
 and medical view of menopause   35
 at work   127–48
 cessation of menses   87–9
 dual role of   131, 138, 143–4
 family changes associated with   81
 fear of becoming old   89
 images of menopause   28
 importance of paid work   129–32
 loss of control over the body   90–1
 menopause as the end of something   87–93
 positive/negative changes in   81–2, 153–4
 self-care for   37
 social changes   91–3
 unconcerned by changes in themselves   80–1, 82
 views on menopause   81, 82–3
 work performance evaluation   131–2, 135–7
 work stories   132–5
 see also mothers; single midlife women
mind–body divide   73–4
mind out of control   52–3, 123, 152
'mind over matter' approach to managing health   155–6
misery during menopause   42
moods   120, 121
'Mother Nature'   160, 171, 181
motherhood   75
mothers
 and daughters' information about menopause   85–6
 becoming like mother   72, 89
 contributing positive attitudes to menopause   83–6
 daughters' assuming similar experience to   84
 lack of treatment for menopause   93–4, 95
 support from   143
myths   32

natural
 menopause as natural   36, 40, 41, 92
 remedies *see* alternative therapies; herbal remedies
natural risk
 family medical history as   156–8
 unavoidability of   169–70
naturopathy   169, 211
networks   139–41
non-English speaking background women   16, 151, 210, 227
nuns   49, 51

oestrogen patch   195
oestrogen replacement therapy *see* HRT
oil of evening primrose, for menopause 30
Ojeda, Linda, *Menopause without Medicine*   38, 63
old age *see* ageing
older women
 attitudes in survey   25–7
 positive memories of menopause   26, 90
osteoporosis
 and menopause   34–5, 101
 health-management strategies   159
 inherited   157, 158
 prevention through HRT   20, 34, 35, 44, 159, 188
 threat of   166, 216
 treatment alternatives to HRT   36
out of sorts   111–12
overweight   111, 112, 113

paid work *see* work
painful menstrual symptoms   50–1
Pap smear   18, 115, 149, 157, 162
 beliefs about   163
 negative experiences over   165
 routine testing   165–6
part-time work, social disapproval of   128–9
patriarchal medical profession *see* male-dominated medical profession

perception of the body 64–73
periods *see* menstruation
personal behaviour, as unnatural health risk 158–60
personal growth 154
personal health management, in midlife 153–4
personal satisfaction 130
pharmaceutical companies 44, 182, 193
physical attractiveness 67, 68–9, 75
physical/physiological decline 152–3, 155, 209
  see also ageing
physical work 97, 107
plastic surgery 37
popular literature
  images of menopause 3, 32–47, 94
  see also magazines
popular texts 37–9
  alternative health model to manage menopause 42–3, 44–6
  approaches to menopause 39–43
  biomedical model to manage menopause 42, 43–4
  feminist approach in 45
  medical bias in 40
  women's use of information in 46–7
power and authority
  of community health carers 218–20
  of medical carers 177, 178, 187–9
pre-menopausal women, thoughts on menopause 19
pregnancy
  ambivalence with 66
  and birthing classes 102
  positive experiences of 51
  through lack of sex education 65
premature ageing 182
premenstrual syndrome 215
premenstrual tension 53, 58
private interviews 3
progesterone 44, 46, 64, 138
psychological decline *see* mental decline
psychosocial stresses during midlife 41

puberty 102

QSR NUD•IST software 7–8, 15, 78–9, 84, 94
qualitative data 2, 7–8
quantitative data 2
questionnaires 5, 6, 14
questions, and perception of risk 7

Reitz, R. 43
relationships
  and menopause 98–9, 100
  and sexuality 67–8, 69, 74, 75, 142–3
  between medical carers and women patients 177, 183–5, 187–9, 192–3, 198
  between women and community carers 211–15
  with men outside marriage 56–7, 61
  see also family
researchers 11–12, 13, 48, 100–3, 149–50, 226–7
respondents
  family, cultural and economic context 15–16
  health and health care status 16–18
  menopausal status 18–19
  use of health professionals 18
responsibility for own health 36, 37, 217–24
  see also self-care
risk perception project 7, 149–170
rural community health care, menopause workshop 221–3
rural medical practice 183–4
rural women, lack of social friendships at work 140–1

same-sex schools 65
samples
  for project as a whole 2–6, 14–16
  for risk perception study 150–1
  for single midlife women study 48–9
  for survey 4–5, 48–9, 150–1
  menopausal status 18–19, 20

representativeness 15–17
screening 17–18, 162–7
  avoidance of 164
  disease threat as motivation for 166–7
  negative experiences of 165
  perceived as prevention 163–4
  routinisation of 164–6
  survey results 162–3
self-care 37, 45, 71, 216
sensitive issues, surveys 6–7
sex and power 68, 69
sex education, lack of 65
sexual body
  attractiveness of the 68–9
  understanding of the 65
sexual desire 61–2, 68, 71, 91, 134
sexuality
  and HRT 61–2, 63–4, 182
  and menopause 101
  and relationships 67–8, 69, 74, 142–3
  and sterilisation 57
Shreeve, C. M. 40
single midlife women 48–76
  controlling the body 54–62
  listening to the body 62–4
  making the body work 50–4
  population sample 48–9
  reflection on pre-menopausal/ pre-midlife body 49–50
  viewing the body 64–73
single women, studies 3, 48–76
sleep problems 109, 114
  see also tiredness
slim body 71
smoking 71, 158
social attitudes towards menopause 28–31
social changes of midlife 91–3
social factors in care of the menopausal woman 180
social life 139–40
social support through work 139–40
social transitions 103
sources of information 33–47, 204, 215–18
  see also specific sources, e.g.

magazines
status passage 86–7, 88–9
stereotypes of menopause 1, 25–9
  'crazy' image of 41–2
  depiction by physicians 173, 177
  rejection of 25, 31
sterilisation 54, 56, 56–7, 88
stress incontinence 216
stresses
  and menopause 41, 132
  during midlife 155
study, as distraction from work and family 144
support services 229
survey, large-scale
  background to 13–14
  data handling 7
  design 5–6, 14–15
  findings 8–9, 16–31
  population 15–16
  researchers' concerns 14
surveying on sensitive issues 6–7
symptoms of menopause
  awareness of 51, 101–2, 105, 126
  discussing openly 30
  emphasis on 34, 40, 42, 90
  interpretation of by health advisers 58–9
  see also particular symptoms e.g. hot flushes

t'ai chi sessions 222
taking charge 97, 98–100, 144–6, 147, 191
'taking responsibility' for one's health 218–20
team research 1
telephone interviews, with health providers 3, 203–4
texts see popular texts
time
  women's need for 132, 137
  given by medical carers 184
'time out' 9, 96–7, 137, 145, 147
tiredness 58, 62, 114, 123, 131, 136–8
toenails 106
transition
  and ageing 89

and body out of control 90–1
and cessation of menses 87–9
and the empty nest 91–3
and the end of something 87–91
as event or process 104
assumed at menopause 9, 78–9
avoiding 93–4
dictionary definition 77
in menopausal literature 78
when there is none 80–7, 104
transition work 95–100, 133
a women's diary view 105–25
treatments *see* menopausal treatments
trust in healers 167–9
tubal ligation 55–6

uncertainty in midlife 153–4
unnatural health risks
  HRT for control 160–2
  personal behaviour as 158–60
uterine cancer 60, 166
  and HRT 61
  and oestrogen 44

vagina
  discharge 58
  dryness 36, 112, 186
viewing the body 64–73
vitamins for menopause 20, 98
voluntary work 141–2, 145

wellness 209–10
'whole person', community relationship with 211–13
wisdom with age 31
woman's diary 105–25
women
  and biological determinism 66–7
  and work 126–48
  attitude to medical advice 172, 189–95
  family responsibilities 57, 129
  negotiating authority 189–95
  perceptions of midlife 13
  relationship with community carers 211–15
  relationship with doctors 177, 183–5, 188

responsibility for their own health 217, 218–20, 224
right to choose treatment 46, 187–8, 191–3, 211–12
trust in carers 167–70
women doctors 192, 194
women's bodies, and dysfunctions 216
women's health
  and midlife 149–70
  and treatments for symptom relief 155
women's health movement, ideological basis 202
work
  and family 131, 134–5, 138, 142–4, 146, 147
  and home 127–8, 131
  and HRT 64, 138–9
  and managing menopausal symptoms 138–9
  and menopause 83, 98, 126, 132, 137
  and midlife women 126–48
  anger and frustration with 110–11
  as economic necessity 131, 134, 145–6
  as network 139–42
  ceasing, impact on health 133
  choice over working 144–6
  coping with 123, 124, 143–4
  financial rewards of 130–1
  hot flushes at 126–7
  importance of 129–32
  reluctance to return to 117
  see also home; physical work; voluntary work
work performance, evaluation during midlife 131–2, 135–7
workplace flexibility 147
working the body 50–4
written interviews 5, 15

younger women
  fear of ageing 210
  images of menopause 26–7

zest at midlife 102